Health science research

Health Science Research

A handbook of quantitative methods

Jennifer K. Peat BSc, PhD

with

Craig Mellis, MD, BS, MPH, FRACP
Katrina Williams, MBBS, MSc, FRACP, FAFPHM
Wei Xuan, MSc, MAppStat

SAGE Publications
London   Thousand Oaks   New Delhi

First published
by Allen & Unwin
83 Alexander St
Crows Nest NSW 2065
Australia

SAGE Publications Ltd
6 Bonhill Street
London EC2A 4PU

SAGE Publications Inc
2455 Teller Road
Thousand Oaks, California 91320

SAGE Publications India Pvt Ltd
32, M-Block Market
Greater Kailash – I
New Delhi 110 048

British Library Cataloguing in Publication data

A catalogue record for this book is
available from the British Library

ISBN 0 7619 7402 4 (hbk)
ISBN 0 7619 7403 2 (pbk)

Library of Congress catalog record available

Index compiled by Russell Brooks
Typeset in 11/12.5pt Goudy by Midland Typesetters, Maryborough, Victoria
Printed in Singapore by South Wind Productions

FOREWORD

Such excitement awaits the person doing research! It is an experience that is hard to describe, but it has to do with the delight of discovery, of having 'gone where no-one has gone before' and of having something to say that is unique. Of course, there's an awful lot of sheer drudgery: after every good meal there's the washing up! And the research person needs to be endowed with a keen competitive spirit and persistence, and also with a willingness to confront mistakes, to tolerate failed hypotheses, to see one's bright ideas hit the dust, to be wrong, and to recognise it. So besides being exhilarating, research can be boring, depressing and difficult!

What makes for good research? It certainly helps to have a research question that excites you. Beyond that there is a need for money to do the work, a good team to support you, and others to be firmly critical so that mistakes are detected early and false leads are abandoned before you become too fond of them to say good-bye. The architecture of the research is also critical and it is here that this book should prove its worth beyond diamonds.

The research process, beginning with the confirmation that your research question really IS new, that it hasn't been answered ages ago or that you have not been gazumped while you were thinking about it, leads through careful sketched plans to choosing the appropriate measures, and so forth. The research methods described in this book focus on questions that require you to go into the community, either the community of patients or the community of the walking well, to obtain your answers. The research methods described are directed at fundamentally epidemiological and clinical questions and so are quantitative, medically orientated and reductionist. This form of research is one that is used to investigate the causes of health problems and to give answers that enable medical and other interventions to be designed for prevention or alleviation. This approach does not include qualitative research methods that provide answers to questions that have to do with attitudes, feelings and social constructs. These forms of research require different methods.

This book will clearly be a great help to young and, to some extent, experienced research workers, focusing on epidemiological and clinical questions framed either in terms of the broad community or patient groups. I recommend it most warmly to these researchers and for this purpose.

Stephen R Leeder, BSc(Med), MBBS, PhD, FRACP, FFPHM, FAFPHM
Dean
Faculty of Medicine
University of Sydney

CONTENTS

CONTRIBUTORS

Elena Belousova MSc

Elena Belousova is a database manager at the Institute of Respiratory Medicine in Sydney. She has extensive experience in relational database administration including data modelling; design and coding of applications for health research; data migration between conflicting formats; and training staff in the use of databases. Elena is currently involved in health-related software development life cycles, including statistical analyses and the interpretation of research results.

Dr Robert Halliday MB BS, BSc(Med), FRACP

Robert Halliday is a practicing Neonatologist and presently head of the Department of Neonatology at The Children's Hospital at Westmead. He has an interest in clinical epidemiology and particularly in medical informatics that has led to involvement in a number of projects within the Children's Hospital as well as with the State health system. Such projects include the establishment of an electronic medical record within the Intensive Care environment, the use of web technology in medicine and the development of clinical databases. His current interest is in marrying the electronic patient record with decision support systems using relational databases.

Professor Stephen Leeder BSc(Med), MBBS, PhD, FRACP, FFPHM, FAFPHM

Stephen Leeder is the Dean of the Faculty of Medicine, Professor of Public Health and Community Medicine of the University of Sydney and a Fellow of the University Senate. He was Foundation Professor of Community Medicine at the University of Newcastle from 1976 to 1985 and Director of the Division of Public Health and Community Medicine at Westmead Hospital in the Western Sydney Area Health Service until the end of 1997. He remains a member of the Western Sydney Area Health Board and chairs its Human Research Ethics Committee and Clinical Policy, Quality and Outcomes Committee. Professor Leeder has an interest in medical education and ethics, health policy communication and strategic approaches to research development and application.

Professor Craig Mellis MD, BS, MPH, FRACP

Craig Mellis is the Professor & Head of the Department of Paediatrics & Child Health at the University of Sydney and also of the Clinical

Health science research

Epidemiology Unit at The Children's Hospital at Westmead, Sydney. He has formal training in paediatric medicine, paediatric respiratory disease, and clinical epidemiology and biostatistics and is actively involved in teaching evidenced based medicine and clinical research methods in undergraduate and postgraduate courses. In addition, he has served on many research grants committees including those of the NH&MRC, Asthma Foundation of NSW and Financial Markets for Child Research. His major research interests include the epidemiology of asthma, particularly the increasing prevalence and potential for primary prevention.

Seema Mihrshahi BSc, MPH

Seema Mihrshahi recently completed a Masters of Public Health at the University of Sydney and is currently the project co-ordinator of a large, multi-centre randomised controlled trail to investigate asthma prevention. She has over six years experience in health research and is competent in most aspects of project management including supervision and training of research staff and students, and designing, implementing and evaluating research protocols. In addition to developing prevention strategies to improve maternal and child health, Seema has a keen interest in methods to improve the health status of people in developing countries.

Associate Professor Jennifer Peat BSc (Hons), PhD

Jennifer Peat has a science background with postgraduate epidemiological and statistical training. She has designed and managed a large number of epidemiological studies on the prevalence of asthma and the effects of environmental risk factors and is currently the Principal Investigator of a large randomised controlled trial to test environmental strategies in the primary prevention of asthma in infancy. In the last four years, she has also been the Hospital Statistician at The Children's Hospital at Westmead, Sydney. In addition to conducting statistical consultations, she is responsible for teaching research methods and scientific writing skills, supervising postgraduate students and helping in the preparation and review of all types of scientific documents.

Brett Toelle DipAppSc (Nursing), BA

Brett Toelle is a research officer at the Institute of Respiratory Medicine in Sydney. He has undergraduate training in nursing and psychology and is currently completing a PhD in psychological medicine in which he is investigating patient adherence with asthma management. Over the last eleven years, he has been responsible for co-ordinating, designing and reporting the data from numerous epidemiological studies.

Dr Katrina Williams MBBS, MSc, FRACP, FAFPHM

Katrina Williams is a paediatrician with public health training. She works at The Children's Hospital at Westmead, Sydney in the Clinical Epidemiology Unit and as a general paediatrician. Her reseqarch interests include general paediatric, neurodevelopmental and psychosocial problems in children and her research experience has included systematic reviews and population-based data collection in these areas. She has been involved in the development of the Cochrane Child Health Field, is an editor for the Developmental, Psychosocial and Learning problems Review Group of the Cochrane Collaboration and was an associate editor and co-author of the recent publication *Evidence-based Paediatrics and Child Health.*

Wei Xuan MSc, MAppStat

Wei Xuan completed his Master of Science in the Department of Mathematics, Peking University and his Master of Applied Statistics at Macquarie University, Sydney. He is currently a biostatistician with the Institute of Respiratory Medicine, University of Sydney and has a special interest in statistical techniques that apply in epidemiology and medical research, including methods for analysing longitudinal data, repeated measures data and multivariate data.

INTRODUCTION

In selecting evidence for any health care practice, the only studies of value are those that have been carefully designed and implemented. Inevitably, these will be the studies that adhere to the highest standards of scientific practice. There is no such thing as a perfect research study, but some studies have more inherent limitations that lead to more profound effects on the results than others. However, all well designed studies have the potential to contribute to existing evidence even though they may not provide definitive results. Under such circumstances, a small study well done may be better than no study at all.[1]

In health research, a merging of the sciences of epidemiology and clinical studies has led to better information about the effectiveness of health practices. Epidemiology is the study of populations in which prevalence (incidence, surveillance, trends) and risk factors for disease (aetiology, susceptibility, association) are measured using the best available methods. Many research methods were first established in this discipline but are now applied widely in clinical settings in order to measure the effectiveness of new treatments, interventions and health care practices with both accuracy and precision. Thus, clinical epidemiology has emerged as a research practice in its own right that can be used to develop reliable diagnostic and measurement tools, to minimise possible sources of error such as bias and confounding, and to report research findings in a scientifically rigorous way. It is also important that any research study has sufficient statistical power to ensure that the results have not arisen by chance and are as precise as possible. Properly conducted research studies that use these methods are able to provide the most reliable evidence of the effects of health care practices and, as such, are a fundamental requirement of evidence-based practice.

This book provides an overview of the essential features of the methods that require careful consideration at all points in the planning, execution or appraisal of a quantitative research study. We have included checklists for a number of research processes including critical appraisal, study design, data management, data analysis and preparing a funding application. In addition, we have provided information and examples of the many methodological issues that must be considered. We hope that this information will help all researchers who are striving to answer questions about effective health care to obtain research funding and to conduct studies of the highest scientific quality. We also hope that this information will be of value to all health care practitioners who need to critically appraise the literature in order to make decisions about the care of their patients. This is essential because only the research studies that aspire to a high scientific standard can be helpful in developing high standards of health care in clinical practice.

Glossary

Term	Meaning
Prevalence	Proportion of a population who have a disease at any one point in time
Incidence	Number of new cases of disease in a population in a specified time period
Aetiology	A descriptor of the processes that cause disease
Bias	Systematic difference between the study results and the truth
Confounding	Process by which the study design leads to a 'mixing' together of the effects of two or more risk factors
Validity	Extent to which an instrument accurately measures what we want it to measure
Repeatability	Accuracy with which a measurement can be replicated

1

REVIEWING THE LITERATURE

Reviewing the literature

Reviewing the literature

The objectives of this chapter are to understand:
- how critical appraisal is used;
- the role of systematic reviews;
- the process of Cochrane reviews; and
- how to facilitate evidence-based practice.

Improving health care delivery

Two essential components in the process of delivering high quality health care are the availability of scientifically valid research studies and the practice of good critical appraisal skills in order to select the most appropriate evidence. Critical appraisal skills are essential for helping to decide whether published research is of a sufficiently high quality to indicate that changes in health practice are required. In this process, the disciplines of critical appraisal and research methods both complement and overlap one another because critical appraisal is a process that helps to identify and foster research studies that use methods of the highest scientific integrity.

Glossary

Term	Meaning
Critical appraisal	Application of rules of scientific evidence to assess the validity of the results of a study
Systematic review	Procedure to select and combine the evidence from the most rigorous scientific studies
Evidence-based practice	Patient care based on the evidence from the best available studies

High quality evidence of health care practices can only be acquired through the implementation of accurate research methods at all stages of a research study, especially the critical stages of study design, data collection and data management, statistical analyses and the interpretation and presentation of the findings. The fundamental issues that must be considered in collecting accurate research data are shown Table 1.1.

Table 1.1 Fundamental issues in research design
Study methods
• merit—type of study
• accuracy—differential and non-differential bias
• randomisation and allocation concealment
• blinding—single or double
• confounding—control in design or analyses
• precision—validity and repeatability of tools
• stopping rules—reducing type I errors
• sample size—statistical power and accuracy
Analysis
• data management
• interim analyses
• statistical and reporting methods
Interpretation
• generalisability
• clinical importance
• level of evidence

Critical appraisal

Scientific merit

Critical appraisal, which is the process used to evaluate the scientific merit of a study, has become an essential clinical tool. The fundamental skills of appraisal are to ask questions about whether a reported association between an intervention or exposure and a health outcome is causal or can be explained by other factors such as chance, bias or confounding. This approach is essential because we can only have confidence in results that could not have arisen by chance, are not affected by bias or confounding, and are not influenced by the statistical methods chosen to analyse the data.

Critical appraisal skills are essential for making decisions about whether to change clinical practice on the basis of the published literature, and for making decisions about the most important directions for future research. In judging an article as valuable evidence, the conclusions reached must be justified in terms of the appropriateness of the study methods used and the validity of the results reported. Judging these merits comes from a sound understanding of the limitations and the benefits of different research methods.

Table 1.2   Steps for critical appraisal
❑ Identify hypothesis
❑ Identify study design
❑ Note criteria for subject selection and sample size
❑ Identify sources of bias
❑ Consider possible effects of confounding
❑ Appraise statistical methods
❑ Consider whether results are statistically significant and/or magnitude is of clinical importance
❑ List strengths and weaknesses
❑ Decide whether conclusion is warranted

Using critical appraisal to prioritise research

A valuable aspect of critical appraisal is that the process can help to prioritise new research by highlighting gaps in knowledge and inadequacies in existing studies. This is important because, at best, poor studies cannot provide answers to questions about the effectiveness of practices but, at worst, they can be misleading. The process of critical appraisal can also provide a formalised system of peer review before published results are considered for incorporation into clinical practice. By highlighting clinical practices for which the evidence of efficacy or effectiveness is poor, the process of critical appraisal also helps to identifiy questions that can only be answered by conducting research studies that are more rigorous than those previously undertaken. The steps for undertaking the critical appraisal of a study that has been designed to address a health care question are shown in Table 1.2.

Critical appraisal checklist

When reviewing an article, it is often useful to have a checklist to help evaluate scientific merit. The checklist shown in Table 1.3 provides a short list of questions to ask when reviewing a journal article for research purposes. Other critical appraisal checklists for more specialised purposes are available. For example, an evaluation method has been developed that ranks studies into five levels of evidence according to the risk of bias.[1] Many journals also provide their own checklists and formats that have to be followed when submitting or reviewing articles and the *British Medical Journal* has excellent checklists for writers, statisticians and reviewers that can be accessed through its website. In addition, other question lists[2,3] and checklists[4-9] provide specific questions that should be asked when deciding whether the evidence reported in an article should be applied in a specific clinical practice.

Not all questions in Table 1.3 apply to all studies—the list is put forward as core questions that can be abbreviated, amended or supplemented according to requirements. The terms and concepts used in the checklist are described in later chapters.

Table 1.3　Checklist of questions for critical appraisal

Introduction
❏ What does this study add to current knowledge?
❏ What are the study aims or what hypotheses are being tested?
Study design
❏ What type of study design has been used?
❏ What are the inherent strengths and weaknesses of this design?
❏ Are the methods described in enough detail to repeat the study?
Subjects
❏ Are the characteristics of the study sample described in detail?
❏ What are the selection methods, including the exclusion/inclusion criteria?
❏ Are the subject numbers adequate to test the hypothesis?
❏ What is the generalisability of the results?

Cont'd

Table 1.3 Cont'd   Checklist of questions for critical appraisal

Measurements
❑ Are the validity and repeatability of the measurements described?
❑ Are the outcome measurements clinically relevant?

Minimisation of bias
❑ What was the response rate?
❑ What is the profile of the refusers or non-responders?
❑ Were the cases and controls sampled from similar populations?
❑ Were all subjects studied using exactly the same protocol?
❑ Could there be any recall or reporting bias?
❑ Was double blinding in place?

Control of confounding
❑ How was the randomisation and allocation concealment carried out?
❑ Have confounders been measured accurately and taken into account?
❑ Were the study groups comparable at baseline?

Results
❑ What are the outcomes (dependent) and explanatory (independent)
   variables?
❑ Do the results answer the study question?

Reporting bias
❑ Are the statistical analyses appropriate?
❑ Are all of the subjects included in the analyses?
❑ Are confidence intervals and P values given?
❑ Could any results be false positive (type I) or false negative (type II)
   errors?

Discussion
❑ Did the choice of subjects influence the size of the treatment effect?
❑ Are the critical limitations and potential biases discussed?
❑ Can the results be explained by chance, bias or confounding?
❑ Are the conclusions justified from the results presented?
❑ Do the results have implications for clinical practice?

Systematic reviews

Narrative and systematic reviews

Narrative reviews and editorials, which appear regularly in most journals, often selectively quote the literature that supports the authors' points of view. These types of articles are essential for understanding new concepts and ideas. However, it is important that health care is based on systematic reviews that include and summarise all of the relevant studies that are available.

Systematic reviews use highly developed methods for finding and critically appraising all of the relevant literature and for summarising the findings. The process of systematic review involves progressing through the prescribed steps shown in Table 1.4 in order to ensure that the review is relevant, comprehensive and repeatable. Once articles have been selected, their results can be combined using meta-analysis. By combining the results of many studies, the precision around estimates of treatment effects and exposure risks can be substantially improved.[10]

Table 1.4   Steps for undertaking a systematic review
❑ Define outcome variables
❑ Identify intervention or exposure of interest
❑ Define search strategy and literature databases
❑ Define inclusion and exclusion criteria for studies
❑ Conduct search
❑ Review of studies by two independent observers
❑ Reach consensus about inclusion of studies
❑ Conduct review
❑ Pool data and conduct meta-analysis
❑ Submit and publish final review

Many systematic reviews have been restricted to the inclusion of randomised controlled trials, although this concept has been relaxed in some areas where such trials cannot be conducted because of practical or ethical considerations. In health areas where there have been few randomised controlled trials, other formal systems for incorporating alternative study designs, such as prospective matched pair designs, are being developed.[11] In terms of summarising the results, this is not a problem because the methods of combining odds ratios from each study into a meta-analysis[12, 13] can also be applied to studies with a less rigorous design.[14]

Cochrane collaboration

The Cochrane collaboration has developed into an important international system of monitoring and publishing systematic reviews. Archie Cochrane was an epidemiologist who, in the late 1970s, first noted that the medical profession needed to make informed decisions about health care but that reliable reviews of the best available evidence were not available at that time. Cochrane recognised that a systematic review of a series of randomised controlled trials was a 'real milestone in the history of randomised controlled trials and in the evaluation of care'. Since that time, this has become the 'gold standard' method of assessing evidence for health care in that it is the method that is widely accepted as being the best available.

Health science research

In 1993, the Cochrane collaboration was established in recognition of Cochrane's insights into the need for up-to-date reviews of all relevant trials in order to provide good health care. Cochrane also recognised that to have ongoing value, reviews must be constantly updated with any new evidence and must be readily available through various media.[15]

Since being established, the Cochrane collaboration has quickly grown into an international network. The collaboration is highly organised with several Internet websites from which the latest information can be accessed in the form of pamphlets, handbooks, manuals, contact lists for review groups and software to perform a review. Many regional Cochrane centres throughout the world can also be contacted via the Internet. Currently, the aims of the Cochrane collaboration are to prepare, maintain and disseminate all systematic reviews of health care procedures. In addition, the collaboration can direct better methods for future research, for example by recommending the inclusion of outcomes that should be measured in future studies.[16]

Cochrane library

Once complete, all Cochrane reviews are incorporated into the Cochrane Database of Systematic Reviews that is disseminated through the Cochrane library. Because of the wide dissemination of information and the process of registering titles and protocols before the final review is complete, any duplication of effort in planned reviews is easily avoided. To be included in a review, the methods used in a trial must conform with strict guidelines, which usually includes randomisation of subjects to study groups and the inclusion of a control group.

The Cochrane database contains completed systematic reviews and approved protocols for reviews that are in progress. The first database was released in 1995 and, since then, the number of reviews has increased substantially. Some Internet sites provide free access to the Cochrane database so that completed reviews are readily accessible to all establishments where appropriate computer equipment is available.

Cochrane review groups

The organisation of the Cochrane collaboration comprises a tiered structure that includes review groups, method working groups and centres. A *Cochrane review group* is a network of researchers and/or clinicians who share an interest in a particular health problem and who provide their own funding. Clinicians and researchers who have an interest in conducting a review of a specific topic first approach the relevant review group to register the title of their review. The next step involves the submission of a protocol, which the review group critically appraises and then asks the authors to amend. Once a protocol is approved, the authors undertake the review by carrying out systematic searches for relevant trials, rating each trial for relevance and quality, assembling and summarising the results, and drawing conclusions of how the net result should be applied in health care. The submitted review is then critically appraised by the review group and amended by the authors before being published as part of the Cochrane library. The authors responsible for a review are also responsible for updating their review each time more information becomes available.

Review groups, who are coordinated by an editorial team, synthesise review modules into the Cochrane database. To support review groups, *method working groups* are responsible for developing sound methods for establishing evidence, synthesising the results and disseminating the reviews. *Cochrane centres* share the responsibility for managing and co-ordinating the collaboration. These centres maintain a register of all involved parties and of all reviews, help to establish review groups and are responsible for developing policies, protocols and software to promote the undertaking of reviews and their use.

Undertaking a Cochrane review

The Cochrane collaboration is based on the principles of encouraging the enthusiasm and interests of clinicians and researchers, minimising duplication of effort, avoiding bias and keeping up to date. The aims of the scheme are to provide volunteer reviewers with the encouragement, skills and supervision that are needed to complete the task to the standard required. The Cochrane collaboration helps its reviewers by providing documents, organising workshops and developing software for summarising the results. The basic principles of the collaboration are shown in Table 1.5.

Table 1.5 Methods used by the Cochrane collaboration to promote high standards of review
• address specific health problems • train experts in the review process • provide a network of people with common interests • avoid duplication of literature reviews • teach efficient search strategies • conduct meta-analyses

There is a common perception that the process of undertaking a Cochrane review is by 'invitation only'. However, anyone, regardless of their position, can volunteer to conduct a review simply by identifying a clinical problem that has not been reviewed previously and by registering their proposed review title with a regional review group. The people who have undertaken Cochrane reviews encompass a wide range of professions including clinicians, health care practitioners, consumers, nurses and research scientists.[17] Information about the collaboration is available in both electronic and printed forms. Anyone interested in learning more should contact their local Cochrane centre.

In recent years, Cochrane reviews have become an integral part of evaluating the effectiveness of health care processes. However, reliable and informative reviews depend on maintaining up-to-date reviews and on identifying as many relevant studies as possible.[18] In the future, the continuation of the Cochrane review process will be complemented with an ongoing development of the methods to include disease conditions that do not lend themselves to investigation by randomised trials. In turn, this process has the exciting potential to guide decisions about better care and better research across a much broader range of health areas.

Evidence-based practice

Procedures for evidence-based practice

Evidence-based practice is an approach that uses the best scientific evidence available to help deliver the best patient care at both an individual and a population level. Cochrane reviews focus mainly on the evidence from randomised controlled trials. However, evidence-based practice is not restricted to these types of studies but is more encompassing in that it involves tracking down the best evidence that is available about the assessment and management of specific health care problems.[19]

The approach of evidence-based practice is based on the principles that it is better to know, rather than believe, what the likely outcome of any intervention will be.[20] Judgments of likely effectiveness are best achieved by using systematic methods to appraise the literature in order to provide valid answers to specific questions about patient care. This process has developed from the acknowledgement that increasing numbers of research studies are being published that have not been conducted to a sufficiently high standard to warrant the incorporation of their results into clinical care practices. The basic procedures of evidence-based practice, which are summarised in Table 1.6, have been widely reported.[21–23]

In the approach of evidence-based practice, both clinical and research experience is needed in order to frame the questions, interpret the evidence, make decisions about treatment policies and direct relevant research questions and research skills. Using this combined approach, a body of corporate knowledge from many diverse experiences can be synthesised to answer questions about health care.

Table 1.6   Procedures for evidence-based practice
❑ Define the problem ❑ Break the problem down into questions that can be answered formally ❑ Find relevant clinical articles by conducting an effective literature search ❑ Select the best studies ❑ Appraise the evidence using criteria such as validity, repeatability, relevance, study strengths and weaknesses, generalisability, results etc. ❑ Make clinical decisions, review policy and implement the findings ❑ Where information is not available, design and conduct new studies ❑ Evaluate the outcomes of changes in practice

Benefits of evidence-based practice

The benefits of evidence-based practice are shown in Table 1.7. Use of scientific reviews of the evidence to assess the effectiveness of clinical practices increases the likelihood that the benefits for patients will be maximised and the use of health services will be more efficient. These processes are facilitated by ready access to systematic reviews, for example through the Cochrane collaboration, and by the publication of appraisals of studies in journals such as *Evidence-Based Medicine*.

Components of care that can be scrutinised using an evidence-based approach include the usefulness of diagnostic tests and the effectiveness of all medications, treatments or health care interventions. However, any changes to health care practice must also take account of other integral factors such as clinician and patient preferences, cost, risk, quality of life, and ability to provide.[24] Because of this, clinical decision-making will always remain a complex process and evidence-based practice should be seen as a reliable tool that helps to facilitate better health care rather than a definitive process that dictates health care practices.[25, 26]

Table 1.7   Benefits of evidence-based practice
• focuses new research on important or practical issues • can be used to evaluate existing practices or support the implementation of new practices • has the potential to lead to more informative decision making and more effective health care • saves time when systematic reviews are available or when appraisals of studies are published

2

PLANNING THE STUDY

Section 1—Study design

The objectives of this section are to understand:
- the types of study designs used in research;
- the strengths and weaknesses of each type of study design;
- the appropriate uses of different study designs;
- the type of study design needed to answer a research question; and
- the type of study design needed to measure the repeatability of an instrument or the agreement between two different instruments.

Designing a study

In designing your own study and appraising the results of studies conducted by other research groups, it is important to recognise the strengths and the limitations of the different types of study design that can be used. The choice of a particular study design is a fundamental decision in designing a research study to answer a specific research question. Once the study design has been decided, then the confidence with which a hypothesis can be tested, or to which causation can be implied, becomes clearer.

Glossary

Term	Meaning
Study design	Methods used to select subjects, assess exposures, administer interventions and collect data in a research study
Hypothesis	Study question phrased in a way that allows it to be tested or refuted
Informed consent	Voluntary participation of subjects after receiving detailed information of the purposes of the study and the risks involved
Generalisability or external validity	Extent to which the study results can be applied to the target population

General terms to describe studies

In addition to the specific names used to identify the types of studies that are described in this chapter, Table 2.1 shows the general terms that are often used. An important distinction between descriptive and experimental studies is that descriptive studies are the only method for measuring the effects of non-modifiable risk factors, such as genetic history or gender, or exposures to which subjects cannot be allocated, such as air pollutants or environmental tobacco smoke. On the other hand, experimental studies are more powerful in that they can provide information about the effects of manipulating environmental factors such as allergen exposures, behaviours such as exercise interventions or dietary choices, and new treatments and health care interventions such as drug treatments or health care practices.

Table 2.1 General terms to describe research studies	
Term	Features of study
Descriptive, non-experimental or observational studies	• used to describe rates of disease in a specific population or study group • used to describe associations between exposure and disease, i.e. to measure risk factors • can be cohort, case-control, cross-sectional, ecological, a case series or a case report • can be quantitative or qualitative • often used to generate rather than test hypotheses
Experimental studies	• used to test the effect of a treatment or intervention • can be randomised or non-randomised trials • can also be case-control and cohort studies that are used to test the effect of an exposure when a randomised controlled trial cannot be used
Clinical trials	• used to demonstrate that a new treatment is better than no treatment, better than an existing treatment or equivalent to an existing treatment
Quantitative studies	• studies in which the data can be analysed using conventional statistical methods
Qualitative studies	• used to gain insight into domains such as attitudes or behaviours • information is collected using unstructured open-ended interviews or questions that cannot be analysed using conventional statistical methods • the subject and not the researcher determines the content of the information collected • useful for generating hypotheses
Methodological studies	• used to establish the repeatability or validity of research instruments

Studies that have outcome information that is collected over a period of time are often described as being either retrospective or prospective studies. However, these terms can be applied to data collected in all types of studies. In the past, case-control and cross-sectional studies have often been called 'retrospective' studies whereas cohort studies and randomised controlled trials have been called 'prospective' studies. This nomenclature is misleading because in cohort studies and in clinical trials, both retrospective and prospective data may be collected during the course of the study. For example, by using a questionnaire that asks 'Have you ever had a migraine headache?' retrospective information is collected, whereas a study in which subjects are called once a week and asked 'Do you have a headache today?' collects information using a prospective approach.

Glossary

Term	Meaning
Retrospective data	Data collected using subjects' recall about illnesses or exposures that occurred at some time in the past or collected by searching medical records
Prospective data	Data collected about subjects' current health status or exposures as the study progresses

Order of merit of studies

In general, the study design that is chosen must be appropriate for answering the research question and must be appropriate for the setting in which it is used. The order of merit of different study types for assessing association or causation is shown in Table 2.2. The placing of a systematic review above a randomised controlled trial really depends on the quality of the systematic review and the scope of the randomised controlled trial. Because of methodological differences, a meta-analysis of the results of a number of small randomised controlled trials may not always agree with the results of a large randomised controlled trial.[1] Obviously, a meta-analysis of the results from a number of small studies in which the methods have not been standardised cannot be considered better evidence than the results from a large, multicentre randomised controlled trial in which bias is reduced by carefully standardising the methods used in all centres.

Table 2.2 Ability of studies in terms of relative strength for assessing causation or association

Order of merit	Type of study	Alternative terms or subsets
1	Systematic review or Randomised controlled trials	Meta-analysis Effectiveness and efficacy trials Equivalence studies Cross-over trials
2	Cohort studies	Longitudinal studies Follow-up studies
3	Non-randomised clinical trials	Pragmatic trials Patient preference studies Zelen's design Comprehensive cohort studies
4	Case-control studies	Matched case-control studies Trials with historical controls Open trials
5	Cross-sectional studies	Population studies
6	Ecological studies	
7	Case reports	

It is difficult to place qualitative studies in this hierarchy because they use a completely different approach. In some situations, qualitative data can uncover reasons for associations that cannot be gained using quantitative methods.

There is also another class of studies called *methodological studies* that are designed to measure the repeatability or validity of an instrument, the agreement between two methods or the diagnostic utility of a test. In such studies, more precise results are obtained if a large random sample with wide variability is enrolled. Bias will occur if subjects are chosen specifically on the basis of the presence or absence of disease so that potential 'false negative' or 'false positive cases' are effectively excluded.

Glossary

Term	Meaning
Outcome variable	Measurement used to describe the primary illness indicator being studied
Exposure	A suspected harmful or beneficial effect being studied
Association	Relation between the exposure and outcome variables
Causation	Direct relation between an exposure variable and the disease that this causes
Risk factor	Exposure factor that is associated with the disease outcome
Confounder	Nuisance variable whose effect is a result of selection bias and must be minimised
Prognostic factor	Factor that predicts that a disease or outcome will develop

Efficacy, effectiveness, efficiency and equivalence

Initially, the safety and effects of using a new treatment are usually established in animal models and then in a small group of volunteers who may not necessarily have the disease that the new drug is intended to treat (Phase I studies). Phase I studies should only ever be used for ensuring that it is safe and feasible to use a new treatment in the community.

Glossary

Term	Meaning
Phase I studies	Initial trial of a new treatment to assess safety and feasibility in a small group of volunteers
Phase II studies	Clinical trials to measure efficacy in a group of patients with the disease
Phase III studies	Large randomised controlled trials or multicentre studies to measure effectiveness or equivalence
Phase IV studies	Post-marketing surveillance to measure rare adverse events associated with a new treatment

Following this, a clinical trial is usually conducted in a larger group of patients to establish *efficacy* under ideal clinical conditions (Phase II studies). Efficacy is a measure of whether an intervention does more good than harm under ideal circumstances.[2] In such studies, a placebo control group may be used so that this type of study can only be conducted for new treatments that have not previously been tested in the target population.

Glossary

Term	Meaning
Efficacy	Effect of treatment under ideal conditions in a research trial
Effectiveness	Effect of treatment in routine clinical practice or in the community
Equivalence	Extent to which a new treatment is equivalent to an existing treatment
Efficiency	Relation between the amount of resources needed to conduct a study and the results achieved
Equipoise	Uncertainty of value of a treatment
Placebo	Sham treatment that has no effect and which subjects cannot distinguish from the active treatment

In studies of efficacy, high-risk patients who are carefully diagnosed and who are likely to adhere to the new treatment regimen are often selectively enrolled. Because of the nature of the study, physicians are usually required to follow a carefully developed protocol and the patients receive regular and more personalised attention from the research team than is usually provided to patients in a community setting. New treatments have to be first tested in this way because if they are not efficacious under these conditions, they will not be effective under less ideal conditions.[3]

Once safety and efficacy are established, a more rigorous full-scale evaluation can be undertaken in larger groups of subjects in order to obtain a more definitive measure of *effectiveness or equivalence* (Phase III studies). Studies of effectiveness, that is the effect of the treatment or intervention when used in the general community or in routine clinical practice, are established in a broader, less controlled setting.[4] These types of studies provide a measure of whether an intervention does more good than harm under the usual circumstances of health care practice in which factors such as misdiagnosis and poor patient compliance are more common. In assessing effectiveness, a new treatment or intervention is usually compared with the effects of current 'best-practice' health care methods.

The logical steps in testing whether an intervention or a treatment is beneficial are shown in Table 2.3.

Table 2.3 Sequence of studies to test a new treatment or intervention	
Type of study	Purpose
Case series and case reports Pilot studies Open label clinical trials Trials with historical controls	To measure appropriateness and feasibility
Cross-sectional studies Cohort studies Case control studies Ecological studies	To measure associations between exposures and outcomes
Clinical trials, preferably randomised and with a control group	To measure efficacy or equivalence and to assess common side effects
Community trials Public health interventions	To measure effectiveness, including cost, and to assess infrequent adverse events

Efficiency is a measure of the resources that are needed to apply a new treatment or intervention. Efficiency studies are often described as cost-effectiveness or cost-benefit studies because their purpose is to measure whether a new intervention is worth its cost in terms of the time or resources that are needed for its administration. The term 'efficiency' is also used when considering the amount of resources needed to conduct a study and, in this context, the cost of conducting the study is usually balanced against the level of evidence collected.

Equivalence studies are designed to show that a new treatment is equivalent to an existing treatment in terms of both its efficacy and the potential for harmful effects associated with its use. An equivalence study is usually planned by first defining an acceptable range for the difference in outcome measurements between the new treatment and established treatment groups such that any value in the range is clinically unimportant. This difference should not encompass an unacceptable risk. Equivalence is then established if the confidence interval around the difference measured between groups is within the defined range.

In equivalence studies, a large sample size is usually needed to avoid the result being ambiguous and thus inconclusive. If the sample size in an equivalence trial is too small, neither equivalence nor difference between the treatments will be established.[6, 7] However, decisions about the size of the difference between treatments that is required to demonstrate equivalence depends on a clinical judgment about the severity and the consequences of the illness condition, and therefore on the size of differences between the outcome measurements that is acceptable.

Randomised controlled trials

Randomised controlled trials are studies in which the subjects are randomly allocated to a new treatment, to a control group or to an existing treatment group. The basic design of a randomised controlled trial with two study groups is shown in Figure 2.1. The control group may be a placebo group or a current best-treatment group. Many studies involve randomisation to three or more treatment groups to compare more than one treatment or to compare the effects of different treatments in isolation and in combination with one another. In randomised controlled trials, the results are obtained by comparing the outcomes of the study groups.

Figure 2.1   Design of a randomised controlled trial

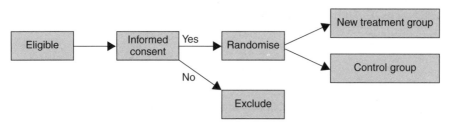

The random allocation of subjects to a treatment group minimises the influences of many factors, including selection bias, known and unknown confounders and prognostic factors, on estimates of efficacy or effectiveness. In addition, measurement bias can be reduced by 'double blinding', that is by ensuring that the researchers who are assessing patient outcomes are unaware of the group status of the subjects and by ensuring that the subjects are unaware of which treatment they are receiving.

Glossary

Term	Meaning
Selection bias	Inappropriate selection of subjects that leads to an over-estimation or under-estimation of the results
Measurement bias	Error that results when an instrument consistently under- or over-estimates a measurement
Misclassification bias	Inaccurate random or directional classification of the outcome or the exposure being investigated

Randomised controlled trials can be used to test the efficacy, effectiveness or equivalence of treatments and to test other health care practices and intervention strategies. Of all study designs, randomised controlled trials provide the highest level of evidence for the effects of an intervention and for causation. Examples of the strengths and limitations of three randomised controlled trials that have been used to measure efficacy, effectiveness and equivalence are shown in Examples 2.1, 2.2 and 2.3.

Example 2.1 Randomised controlled trial to measure efficacy Lebel et al. Dexamethasone therapy for bacterial meningitis[8]	
Characteristic	Description
Aims	To evaluate the efficacy of dexamethasone therapy in children with bacterial meningitis as an adjunct to antimicrobial therapy
Type of study	Double-blinded placebo controlled randomised trial
Subjects	200 infants and older children admitted to hospital with meningitis
Treatment groups	The four study groups comprised two schedules for administering cefuroxime (antimicrobial therapy) each with saline (placebo) or dexamethasone (experimental treatment) as follows: Group 1: regular cefuroxime plus saline (n=49) Group 2: regular cefuroxime plus dexamethasone (n=51) Group 3: staged cefuroxime plus saline (n=49) Group 3: staged cefuroxime plus dexamethasone (n=51)
Randomisation	Computer generated list of random therapy assignments
Outcome measurements	Concentrations of glucose, lactate and protein in cerebrospinal fluid; time to become afebrile; death or severe hearing loss
Statistics	Fisher's exact test; ANOVA with Bonferroni post-hoc tests
Conclusion	• total days with fever, time to resolution of fever and hearing impairment all significantly reduced in both active treatment (dexamethasone) groups • dexamethasone is a beneficial treatment for infants and children with bacterial meningitis, particularly in preventing deafness
Strengths	• confounders (gender, ethnicity, duration of illness, clinical score) evenly balanced between groups • evidence of efficacy helps resolve contradictory results from previous, less rigorous studies
Limitations	• equal numbers in study groups suggests a method other than simple randomisation was used • rate of recruitment to study not given therefore generalisability not known • sample size too small to measure efficacy in terms of less common outcomes, e.g. prevention of death

Example 2.2   Randomised controlled trial to test the effectiveness of an intervention

Nishioka et al. Preventive effect of bedding encasement with microfine fibres on housedust mite sensitisation[9]

Characteristic	Description
Aims	To investigate whether bedding encasing made from microfine fibres can prevent high-risk infants from becoming sensitised to housedust mite allergens
Type of study	Randomised controlled trial
Sample base	Infants attending an outpatient clinic for allergic symptoms
Subjects	57 infants with atopic dermatitis and positive skin prick tests to food allergens but not to housedust mites randomised to an active (n=26) or control (n=27) group
Randomisation	Randomisation method not stated
Intervention	Encasing of mattresses and doonas of all family members in active group; advice about bedding cleaning to both groups
Outcome measurements	Levels of housedust mite allergens in child's bedding; skin prick tests to housedust mite allergens
Statistics	Chi square tests to compare rates of allergic responses
Results	• Sensitisation to housedust mites was 31% in active group and 63% in control group ($P<0.02$) • Occurrence of wheeze was 11% of active group and 37% of control group ($P<0.05$)
Conclusion	• the intervention significantly reduced housedust mite exposure levels • bedding encasing is effective for preventing sensitisation to housedust mites and early symptoms of wheeze in atopic infants
Strengths	• randomisation would have reduced effects of confounding • similar rates of contact and collection of outcomes data in both groups would have reduced bias • objective exposure measurements collected
Limitations	• independent effects of each part of intervention not known • long follow-up time will be required to determine effect of intervention in reducing the incidence of asthma • sample size may not be large enough to detect future clinically important differences after allowing for loss to follow-up

Example 2.3 Randomised controlled trial to test the equivalence of
treatments for severe asthma

Idris et al. Emergency department treatment of severe asthma. Metered
dose inhaler plus holding chamber is equivalent in effectiveness to
nebuliser[10]

Characteristic	Description
Aims	To investigate the equivalence of administration of bronchodilator by nebuliser or metered-dose inhaler for treating acute asthma in an emergency department
Type of study	Double-blinded, randomised trial
Population	Patients with moderate to severe asthma attending for treatment at two emergency centres
Subjects	35 patients age 10–45 years
Treatment groups	20 patients who received treatment by nebuliser and 15 patients who received treatment by inhaler and placebo treatment by nebuliser
Randomisation	No methods given
Outcome measurements	Lung function measurements (FEV1 and FVC) and airflow limitation (peak expiratory flow rate) as percentage of predicted normal values
Statistics	Student t-tests
Conclusion	• no statistical or clinical important difference in the efficacy of the two treatments was found • the metered dose inhaler delivered a complete dose of bronchodilator more quickly and at no additional cost
Strengths	• patients randomised to treatment groups and objective outcome measurements used • placebo nebuliser treatment incorporated
Limitations	• small sample size precluded estimating differences in equivalence between age, severity and other treatment groups • randomisation with small sample size did not balance prognostic factors equally between groups e.g. use of other medications • equivalence in mild asthmatics not established • differences in outcomes important to patient (time in emergency department, number of treatments to discharge, etc.) not measured

Before subjects are enrolled in a randomised controlled trial, their eligibility in terms of inclusion and exclusion criteria must be ascertained and informed consent must be obtained. Following this, subjects are then randomly allocated to their study group. Although a randomised controlled trial is the most scientifically rigorous method available with which to evaluate a new treatment and the design confers many benefits providing the sample size is adequate, Table 2.4 shows that this method may still have some inherent limitations.

Table 2.4   Strengths and limitations of randomised controlled trials
Strengths
• most scientifically rigorous method for measuring short-term outcomes
• study groups are comparable in regard to confounders, environmental exposures and important prognostic factors
• each subject has an equal chance of being allocated to a treatment or control group
• willingness to participate and other factors that may influence outcome do not influence group allocation
Limitations
• need a very large sample size to measure the effects of infrequent adverse outcomes or beneficial outcomes that are rare events
• unsuitable for subjects with strong treatment preferences
• groups may not be comparable if subjects in the control group are disappointed to receive the current treatment and subjects in the experimental group are pleased to receive the new treatment
• may exclude some types of patients to whom the results will subsequently be applied
• may not be continued for a sufficient period to measure long-term or adverse events

Sample size is a fundamental issue in randomised controlled trials. If only small improvements in the outcome measurements between groups are expected, as may be the case for many chronic diseases, or if the expected outcome occurs infrequently in either group, then a large sample size will be required before these differences achieve statistical significance. This is discussed in more detail in Chapter 4. In many trials, the sample size is not large enough to measure side effects that are serious but occur only rarely.[11] Furthermore, the length of trial may be too short to measure adverse effects that take some time to develop. Because of this, the monitoring of adverse events associated with new treatments is usually undertaken in post-marketing surveillance surveys (Phase IV studies) when large numbers of patients have been using the drug for a long period.

In randomised controlled trials, the quality of the evidence is improved if measurement bias, such as observer or reporting bias, is reduced by using objective outcome measurements and if observers are blinded to the group status of the subjects. The methods that are commonly used to minimise bias in randomised controlled trials are summarised in Table 2.5. Random allocation and efficient allocation concealment practices need to be put in place to prevent the recruiting team having prior knowledge of group allocation. It is also important to collect information about the people who choose not to enter the study in addition to collecting some follow-up information of people who drop out of the study. This information is essential for describing the generalisability of the results and for use in intention-to-treat analyses (see Chapter 7).

Table 2.5   Methods to reduce bias in randomised controlled trials

- efficient randomisation methods that achieve balance in numbers between study groups must be used
- the randomisation method must be concealed from the researchers who are responsible for recruiting the subjects
- double-blinding is used to reduce the effects of expectation on the measurement of outcome data
- objective and clinically important outcome measurements are used
- intention-to-treat analyses are used to report the findings
- a large sample size is enrolled in order to measure effects with precision
- pre-planned stopping rules are administered by an external safety committee
- interim analyses are planned and are conducted by a data monitoring committee who conceal the results from the staff responsible for data collection

---

In studies in which the effectiveness of a treatment or intervention is measured, a group of subjects who have an identifiable disease or medical problem are enrolled. However, in studies in which the effect of a primary prevention is being measured, a group of subjects who are 'at risk' of developing the disease are ideally enrolled before any early signs of the disease have developed. Because nearly all treatments or interventions have some unwanted or harmful effects, the benefits of the study have to be estimated in relation to the associated risks. Also, because a large amount of confidence is placed on randomised controlled trials in the application of evidence-based practice, comprehensive reporting of the methods is essential. The methods and results of many clinical trials have not been adequately reported[12] although guidelines for complete reporting of the study procedures are now available.[13, 14]

Glossary

Term	Meaning
Primary prevention	Treatment or intervention to prevent onset of a disease
Secondary prevention	Treatment of early signs to prevent progression to establishment of a disease
Tertiary prevention	Treatment of symptoms after the disease is established

Placebo controlled trials

The use of a placebo group in a trial always requires careful consideration. A trial may be unethical when subjects in the control group are administered a placebo treatment so that they are denied the current best treatment that has proven effectiveness.[15, 16] In studies in which a placebo treatment is included, the researchers must be in a position of equipoise, that is they must be uncertain about which treatment is 'best' before subjects are enrolled.[17-19]

The main use of placebo controlled trials is to assess the benefits of a new treatment whose effects are not yet known but for which a scientifically rigorous method to assess efficacy is required. The most appropriate application for trials with a placebo group is Phase II studies, that is the initial stages of testing new treatments or health care practices.[20] For example, a new class of drug called leukotriene receptor agonists were first tested as a therapy for asthma against a placebo to ensure that they had a beneficial effect.[21] Now that efficacy is established, effectiveness will need to be compared with other treatments in Phase III and Phase IV studies.

Placebo controlled trials usually have a small sample size and, as such, are an intermediate rather than a definitive step in establishing the efficacy of a new treatment.[22] However, there have been many examples of placebo controlled trials being conducted, some for long periods, even though subjects in the control group were withheld from receiving treatments with an established beneficial effect.[23] On the other hand, trials without a placebo group that are conducted in clinical settings where no 'gold standard' treatment exists may provide misleading results because the 'placebo' effect of treatment cannot be taken into account in the evaluation process.[24, 25]

Pragmatic trials

Pragmatic trials, which are an adaptation of the randomised controlled trial design, are used to assess the effect of a new treatment under the conditions of clinical practice. Thus, pragmatic trials are often used to help decide whether a new treatment has advantages over the best current treatment. In this type of trial, other existing treatments are often allowed, complex treatment methods are often compared and outcome measurements that are patient-orientated, such as quality of life or survival rates, are often used. The processes of recruitment and randomisation are the same as those used in randomised controlled trials but because the difference between the two treatment methods will reflect the likely response in practice, pragmatic trials can only be used to measure effectiveness, and not efficacy.

In pragmatic trials, blinding is not always possible so that bias as a result of subject and observer awareness is more difficult to control. Pragmatic trials are often used to test methods to improve the health care of specific groups of patients and, as such, are designed to help clinicians choose the best treatment for a particular group of patients. However, a large sample size is needed to measure the separate beneficial effects in different groups of patients, or in patients who are using different additional treatments.

An example of a pragmatic trial in which patients were randomised to surgery or to a waiting group is shown in Example 2.4. The strengths of this trial in collecting new information about the effectiveness of the treatment were balanced against the limitations of loss of generalisability because many subjects were not randomly allocated to a study group.

In common with randomised controlled trials, the data from pragmatic trials are analysed by 'intention-to-treat' methods. Intention-to-treat analyses are conducted regardless of changes in treatment and, to be most informative, the outcome measurements must include improvements in patient relevant outcomes, such as quality of life, in addition to objective indicators of improvements in illness, such as biochemical tests.

Example 2.4	Pragmatic trial to measure effectiveness of second eye surgery

Laidlaw et al. Randomised trial of effectiveness of second eye cataract surgery[26]

Characteristic	Description
Aims	To examine the effectiveness of surgery on the second eye following surgery on the first eye
Type of study	Randomised clinical trial
Sample base	807 healthy patients awaiting surgery
Subjects	208 patients who consented to participate
Randomisation	By numbered sealed envelopes in blocks of 20; envelopes generated by researchers not in contact with patients
Outcome measurements	Questionnaire responses about visual difficulties; visual function tests
Statistics	Intention-to-treat between-group comparisons
Conclusion	Second eye surgery marginally improves visual acuity and substantially reduces self-reported visual difficulties
Strengths	• balanced numbers achieved in study groups • confounders (gender, age, symptoms) balanced between groups • careful development and choice of outcome variables • more rigorous methods than previous case studies and uncontrolled trials • good evidence of effectiveness collected
Limitations	• modest consent rate limits generalisability • possible reporting bias by patients not blinded to group status could account for disparity of results between objective outcome (visual acuity) and subjective outcome (self reported visual difficulties)

Health science research

Run-in phases and effects of non-compliance

Run-in phases prior to randomisation in any clinical trial can be useful in that they give the subjects time to decide whether or not they want to commit to the trial, and they give the researchers time to identify non-compliant subjects who may be excluded from the study. Such exclusions have an important impact on the generalisability of the results but they also significantly reduce the dilution of non-compliance on any estimates of effect. The advantage of recruiting subjects who are likely to be compliant is that a smaller sample size and fewer resources are required and therefore the study is more efficient. In addition, because a smaller sample size is required, the completion of the trial and the dissemination of the results are not unnecessarily delayed.

Cross-over trials

In cross-over trials, subjects are randomly allocated to study groups in which they receive two or more treatments given consecutively.[27] In this type of trial, the randomisation procedure simply determines the order in which the subjects receive each treatment. Figure 2.2 shows the simplest type of cross-over trial in which one group receives the new treatment followed by the current best treatment, whilst the other group receives the current best treatment followed by the new treatment.

Figure 2.2   Study design for a cross-over trial

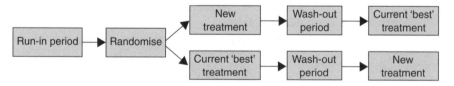

Cross-over trials are most appropriate for measuring the effects of new treatments or variations in combined treatments in subjects with a chronic disease. The advantage of this type of study is that any differences in outcomes between treatments can be measured in the same subjects. Because the outcomes of interest are the within-subject differences, cross-over trials require fewer subjects and therefore are more efficient than randomised controlled trials with parallel groups. A disadvantage of cross-over trials is that bias can occur when the data from subjects who do not go on to the second phase, because they drop out during or after the first treatment period, have to be excluded in the analyses. An outline of a typical cross-over trial is shown in Example 2.5.

Another disadvantage with cross-over trials is that there may be a 'carry-over' effect in subjects who begin the second phase with better health as a result of the first phase. This effect can be minimised with a 'wash-out' period between the treatments. Because of the impact of the wash-out period, the time that is needed for the treatment to have an effect and the time that is needed for the effect to dissipate before the cross-over to the alternative treatment must be carefully considered at the study design stage. The wash-out period must be sufficient to allow the treatment effect to dissipate and the patient must also be able to manage with no treatment during this period.

It is possible to minimise the 'carry-over' effect at the data analysis stage of a cross-over trial. The simplest method is to only use the outcome data collected at the end of each treatment period in the primary data analyses. Another method is to explore whether there is a statistically significant interaction between the treatment sequence and the outcome.[28] However, cross-over trials usually have a small sample size and often do not have the power to explore these types of interactions. In such studies, a subjective judgment about the size of the effect in addition to the statistical significance will need to be made. If an effect seems likely, the analyses can be confined to the first period alone but this approach not only reduces the statistical power but also raises questions about the ethics of conducting a trial with too few subjects to fulfil the study aims.

Glossary

Term	Meaning
Preference group	Group who have self-selected their treatment or who have had their group decided by the researcher
Placebo group	Group receiving a sham treatment that has no effect
Control group	Group with which a comparison is made
Blinding	Mechanism to ensure that observers and/or subjects are unaware of the group to which the subject has been allocated
Randomisation	Allocation of subjects to study groups by chance
Allocation concealment	Concealment of randomisation methods from observers

Example 2.5	Cross-over trial to measure the effectiveness of a treatment

Ellaway et al. Randomised controlled trial of L-carnitine[29]

Characteristic	Description
Aim	To measure the effectiveness of L-carnitine in improving functional limitations in girls with Rett Syndrome
Type of study	Randomised double-blind cross-over trial
Sample base	39 girls with Rett Syndrome ascertained via a national register
Subjects	35 girls who consented to take part
Treatment	Subjects randomised to receive sequential treatments of 8 weeks of L-carnitine, wash-out of 4 weeks then placebo for 8 weeks, or to receive 8 weeks placebo, wash-out for 4 weeks and then L-carnitine for 8 weeks.
Outcome measurements	Behavioural and functional ratings by scores on a 5-point scale; qualitative data collected by semi-structured interview
Statistics	Non-parametric Wilcoxon matched-pairs signed-ranks tests to measure within-subject differences between placebo and active treatment periods
Conclusion	• L-carnitine may be of more benefit to patients with classical Rett Syndrome than to atypical variants • subtle improvements in some patients had a significant impact on families
Strengths	• compliance verified using plasma L-carnitine levels • appropriate study design for estimating the effect of a new treatment on girls with a chronic condition • long wash-out period included • carry-over effect minimised by only using data from the end of each placebo/treatment period in the analyses
Limitations	• 4 institutionalised girls with inconsistent carers had to be omitted from data analyses • validity of outcomes data collected by institution carers not known • blinding may have been incomplete because of fishy body odour and loose bowel actions associated with L-carnitine • outcome measurement scales not responsive enough to detect small changes in functional ability that had an important impact on families

Zelen's design

Zelen's design,[30, 31] which is also called a *randomised consent* design, is a modified randomised controlled trial design in which randomisation occurs before informed consent is obtained, and consent is only obtained from the group who are allocated to receive the experimental treatment. This type of study design is only used in situations in which the new or experimental treatment is invasive and the illness condition is severe, such as in some trials of cancer therapies.

If randomisation to a standard treatment or a placebo group is unacceptable or impossible, then this type of less rigorous clinical trial reduces problems caused by low rates of subject consent. In studies with Zelen's design, subjects are randomised to receive the experimental or standard treatment but only remain in the experimental treatment group if they find it acceptable. Subjects who do not consent to be in the experimental group are assigned to the standard treatment group but their data are analysed as if they were in the experimental group. The design of this type of study is shown in Figure 2.3.

Figure 2.3   Zelen's double randomised consent design

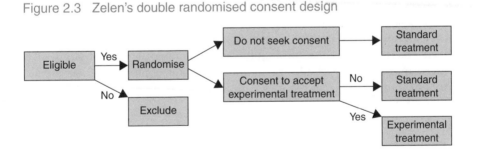

In this type of trial, a subject agrees to receive the experimental treatment only if it is their personal treatment preference or if they have no preference. This study design is especially useful for overcoming the low recruitment rates that often occur when a new type of invasive treatment is being introduced and has the advantages that generalisability and statistical power in terms of subject numbers are maximised. However, this is achieved at the cost of not being able to control for possible confounders.

Glossary

Term	Meaning
Statistical power	Ability of the study to demonstrate an association if one exists or to measure the size of an effect with a specified precision
Precision	Accuracy with which an effect is demonstrated, usually measured by the standard error or the confidence interval around the estimate
Interaction	Ability of two factors to increase or decrease each other's effects, often described by a multiplicative term in regression analyses

Comprehensive cohort studies

A comprehensive cohort study, which is also called a *prospective cohort study with a randomised sub-cohort*, is a study design whereby subjects consent to be randomised or are offered their choice of treatment as shown in Figure 2.4. This study design produces two cohorts of subjects, one that is randomised to a treatment regime and one who self-select their treatment. A comprehensive cohort study design, which is useful when a large proportion of subjects are likely to refuse randomisation, is commonly used in trials such as those in which the results of radiotherapy are compared to surgery as a cancer therapy. An example of a comprehensive cohort study is shown in Example 2.6.

Figure 2.4   Comprehensive cohort study design

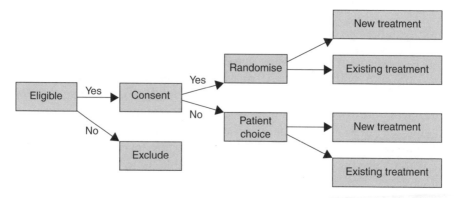

In comprehensive cohort studies, the effects of group allocation on outcome and the association with psychosocial factors can be explored. This study design has an advantage over Zelen's design because all eligible subjects can be included and the subject's freedom of choice is respected. Other more complex types of studies that have both an informed consent and randomised consent group have also been suggested.[32] Comprehensive cohort studies are similar to trials with a preference group in that they only provide supplemental results rather than providing definitive information about the efficacy or effectiveness of a new treatment.

By using randomisation status as an indicator variable in the analysis, it is possible to measure the extent to which results from the small proportion who consent to randomisation can be extrapolated to the larger group with disease. Although this helps to establish the generalisability of the results, the randomised sub-group needs to be large enough to establish a significant effect of treatment in its own right, and the study cannot be a substitute for a well designed randomised controlled trial. Ultimately, an independent randomised controlled trial will still be needed to provide definitive evidence that has broader generalisability.

Example 2.6 Comprehensive cohort study	
Agertoft et al. Effects of long-term treatment with an inhaled corticosteroid on growth and pulmonary function in asthmatic children[33]	
Characteristic	**Description**
Aim	To measure the effects of long-term treatment with inhaled corticosteroids on growth and lung function in asthmatic children
Type of study	Comprehensive cohort study with patient preference groups
Sample base	Children with mild or moderate asthma and no other chronic disease who had attended a clinic for 3 visits over 1 year
Subjects	The cases were 216 children whose parents consented to their taking inhaled corticosteroids for 3–6 years. The controls were 62 children, most of whom were treated with cromoglycate, whose parents did not want them to receive inhaled corticosteroids

Cont'd

Example 2.6 Cont'd   Comprehensive cohort study

Characteristic	Description
Outcome measurements	Growth velocity, weight gain, hospital admissions for asthma, improvement in % predicted FEV1
Statistics	Analysis of variance and regression to measure effects over time
Conclusions	• treatment associated with reduced hospital admission for asthma and improved FEV1 • no difference in growth velocity or weight gain between groups
Strengths	• baseline information collected during a run-in period • results of bias minimised by using a cohort study design and objective outcome measurements • information obtained that was otherwise not available
Limitations	• no randomised group to control for confounders • only supplemental evidence gained

Non-randomised clinical trials

In non-randomised trials, the subject or the researcher decides the group to which subjects are assigned. This type of trial is only appropriate for distinguishing between therapeutic effects and patient preference effects that cannot be measured in a randomised trial. The decision to conduct a non-randomised trial needs careful consideration because a major disadvantage is that the information obtained is only supplemental to evidence of efficacy or effectiveness obtained from a randomised trial. For this reason, non-randomised trials should only be used to answer questions that cannot be addressed using a randomised controlled trial.

The results of trials in which subjects are allocated by personal preference to a new treatment will give very different information to that obtained from randomised controlled trials, although one method does not necessarily give a consistently greater effect than the other.[34] Subjects who participate in different types of trials tend to have quite different characteristics. In randomised trials to evaluate the treatment of existing illnesses, subjects tend to be less affluent, less educated and less healthy whereas the subjects in trials of preventive interventions tend to be the opposite.[35] An advantage of non-randomised trials is that the information gained may have greater generalisability. In randomised trials, the response rate may be low because the inclusion criteria are strict or because large numbers of subjects decline to enrol. Also, subjects who agree to enrol because they will obtain a new and otherwise unavailable treatment are more likely to drop out if they are randomised to the standard care group. These factors may cause significant selection bias that detracts from the generalisability of the results.[36]

Selection bias is less likely to occur in trials with a preference group because patients are more likely to consent to enrol in the study. However, non-randomised allocation naturally creates a greater potential for allocation bias to distort the results because important confounders may not be balanced evenly between the study groups. In addition, compliance with the new treatment or intervention is likely to be higher in the preference group than would occur in a general clinical setting. Because a preference group will provide information about the effect of a treatment that is chosen by subjects who already believe it will help them, the results may suggest that the treatment is more effective than results obtained from a trial in which allocation is random.

Although many subjects prefer to make their own choices about factors such as diet, self-medication, monitoring and trial entry, the ways in which such preferences alter outcomes are not easily measured and are not always clear. It is possible to reduce bias as a result of patient preference with the use of objective outcome measurements and blinded observers. If randomised and non-randomised groups are included and if the sample size is large enough, the extent of the bias can also be estimated by analysing the randomised and personal preference groups separately and then comparing the results.

Open trials

Open trials, which are often called *open label trials*, are clinical studies in which no control group is enrolled and in which both the patient and the researcher are fully aware of which treatment the patient receives. These types of trials only have a place in the initial clinical investigation of a new treatment or clinical practice (Phase I studies). From an ethical point of view, subjects must understand that the treatment is in a developmental stage and that they are not taking part in a trial that will answer questions of efficacy. In general, open trials are likely to produce results that are over-optimistic because bias in a positive direction as a result of expectation of benefit cannot be minimised.

Cohort studies

Cohort studies, which are sometimes called *prospective studies* or *longitudinal studies*, are conducted over time and are used to describe the natural history or the 'what happens next?' to a group of subjects. In these studies, subjects are enrolled at one point in time and then followed prospectively to measure their health outcomes. The time of enrolment is usually specific, for example at birth when subjects are disease-free or at a defined stage of disease, such as within twelve months of diagnosis. As such, cohort studies are usually used to compare the health outcomes of groups of subjects in whom exposures or other attributes are different. The design of a cohort study is shown in Figure 2.5. In such studies, the risk of developing a disease is calculated by comparing the health outcomes of the exposed and unexposed groups.

Figure 2.5   Design of a cohort study

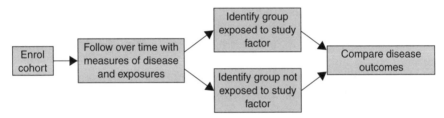

In the study of populations, cohort studies are the only type of study that can be used to accurately estimate incidence rates, to identify risk factors, or to collect information to describe the natural history or prognosis of disease. However, these types of studies are often expensive to conduct and slow to produce results because a large study sample and a long follow-up time are needed, especially if the outcome is rare. Also, cohort studies have the disadvantage that the effects of exposures that change over the study period are difficult to classify and to quantify. On the other hand, these types of studies have the advantage that the effects of risk factors can be measured more accurately than in cross-sectional or case-control studies because the rate of development of a disease can be compared directly in the exposed and non-exposed groups. As a result, cohort studies are the most appropriate study design with which to establish temporal relationships. The desirable features of a cohort study are shown in Table 2.6.

Table 2.6	Desirable features of cohort studies

Subjects
- a random population sample is enrolled as an inception cohort, that is very early in life or at a uniform point in time
- follow-up rates of at least 80% are achieved throughout the study
- the inclusion and exclusion criteria are easily reproducible
- there is good comparability between the subjects who continue or who drop out of the study
- no intervention is applied during the follow-up period
- the follow-up time is long enough for the disease to resolve or develop

Measurements
- more than one source of outcome variable is investigated
- objective outcome measurements are used
- subjective outcomes are assessed by observers who are blinded to the subject's exposure status

Analyses
- analyses are adjusted for all known confounders

In cohort studies, the enrolment of a random sample of the population ensures generalisability and methods to minimise non-response, follow-up and measurement bias are essential for maintaining the scientific integrity of the study. In addition, exposure must be ascertained before the disease or outcome develops and the disease must be classified without knowledge of exposure status. An outline of a cohort study is shown in Example 2.7.

Example 2.7	Cohort study
Martinez et al. Asthma and wheezing in the first six years of life[37]	
Characteristic	**Description**
Aims	To measure the association of symptoms of wheeze in early life with the development of asthma, and to measure risk factors that predict persistent wheeze at age 6 years
Type of study	Prospective cohort study
Sample base	Cohort of 1246 newborns enrolled between 1980–1984
Follow-up period	6 years
Subjects	826 children remaining in cohort
Outcome measurements	Classification by wheeze severity (none, transient, late onset or persistent)

Cont'd

Example 2.7 Cont'd   Cohort study

Characteristic	Description
Explanatory measurements	Respiratory symptoms, maternal asthma, ethnicity, gender, parental smoking
Statistics	Analysis of variance to measure associations; odds ratios to measure risk factors
Conclusions	• Wheeze in early life is associated with low lung function in early life but not with later asthma or allergy • Risk factors associated with persistent wheeze at age 6 are maternal asthma, ethnicity, gender, maternal smoking and a high serum IgE, but not low lung function
Strengths	• large inception cohort enrolled with long follow-up period achieved • some objective measurements used (lung function, serum IgE) • risk factors are measured prospectively, i.e. more accurately • exposure to risk factors was measured before the outcomes developed
Limitations	• moderate follow-up rate may have biased estimates of incidence to some extent and estimates of risk to a lesser extent • information of non-responders is not available • effects of different treatment regimes on outcomes are not known

Case-control studies

In case-control studies, subjects with a disease of interest are enrolled and compared with subjects who do not have the disease. Information of previous exposures is then collected to investigate whether there is an association between the exposure and the disease. Because past exposure information is collected retrospectively, case-control studies often rely on the subject's recall of past events, which has the potential to lead to bias.

The design of a case-control study is shown in Figure 2.6. These types of studies are widely used in research because they are usually cheaper and provide answers more quickly than other types of study design. In case-control studies, the controls are selected independently of the cases, whereas in matched case-control studies each control is selected to match the defined characteristics, such as age or gender, of each case.

Figure 2.6   Case-control study design

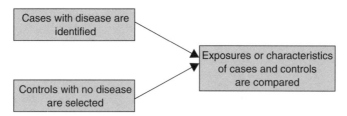

There are many methods of selecting cases and controls.[38, 39] Cases may be chosen to represent either mild or severe disease, or both, but either way the inclusion criteria must be specific. The ideal controls are those who are randomly selected from the same study base or the same population from which the cases are drawn. Although controls may be selected from the same hospital or clinic population as the cases, it is preferable to select from friends, schools or neighborhoods, or ideally from registers such as telephone directories or electoral lists. Whatever the source, the most appropriate controls are subjects who would have been enrolled as cases if they had developed the disease. To increase statistical power, more than one control can be enrolled for each case (see Chapter 4). An example of a case-control study is shown in Example 2.8.

In case-control studies, the results are based on comparing the characteristics, or exposures, of the cases with those of the controls. The risk of disease is often estimated by comparing the odds of the cases having an exposure with the odds of the controls having the same exposure. However, when exposures are reported retrospectively by the subjects themselves, the measurements may be subject to recall bias. Case-control studies cannot be used to infer causation because it is difficult to control for the influence of confounders and for selection bias. Uncontrolled confounding and bias can lead to distorted estimates of effect and type I errors (the finding of a false positive result), especially if the effect size is small and the sample size is large.

Because the results from case-control studies are most useful for generating rather than testing hypotheses about causation, these types of studies are often used in the first stages of research to investigate whether there is any evidence for proposed causal pathways. However, the findings of case-control studies are often overturned in subsequent studies that have a more rigorous scientific design. For example, the results from a case-control study in England suggested that there was a relation between neonatal intra-muscular administration of vitamin K and childhood cancer, with a statistically significant odds ratio of 2.0 (95% CI 1.3, 3.0, $P<0.01$).[40] This result was later overturned in a study that had a more rigorous cohort design and a large sample size, and in which a non-significant odds ratio of 1.0 (95% CI

0.9, 1.2) was found.[41] In this later study, hospital records were used to measure vitamin K exposure in infants born in the period 1973–1989 and the national cancer registry was accessed to measure the number of cases of cancer. These methods were clearly more reliable than those of the case-control study in which self-reported exposures were subject to recall bias.

Nested case-control studies

Nested case-control studies can be conducted within a cohort study. When a case arises in the cohort, then control subjects can be selected from the subjects in the cohort who were at risk at the time that the case occurred. This has the advantage that the study design controls for any potential confounding effects of time.

Nested case-control studies are often used to reduce the expense of following up an entire cohort. The advantage is that the information gained is very similar to the information that would be gained from following the whole cohort, except that there is a loss in precision.

Example 2.8 Case-control study to measure risk factors Badawi et al. Antepartum and intrapartum risk factors for newborn encephalopathy: the Western Australian case-control study[42, 43]	
Characteristic	Description
Aim	To identify predictors of newborn encephalopathy in term infants
Type of study	Population based, unmatched case-control study
Sample base	Births in metropolitan area of Western Australia between June 1993 and September 1995
Subjects	Cases: all 164 term infants with moderate or severe newborn encephalopathy born in described period Controls: 400 controls randomly selected from term babies born during same period as cases
Outcome measurement	Risk of outcome in presence of several measures of exposure
Statistics	Descriptive statistics, odds ratios and 95% confidence intervals
Conclusions	• many causes of newborn encephalopathy relate to risk factors in the antepartum period • intrapartum hypoxia accounts for only a small proportion of newborn encephalopathy • elective caesarean section has an inverse relation with newborn encephalopathy

Cont'd

Example 2.8 Cont'd   Case-control study to measure risk factors

Characteristic	Description
Strengths	• able to investigate all risk factors by avoiding the use of matching and by avoiding the use of presumed aetiological factors in the case definition • controls randomly selected from population and demonstrated to be representative in terms of important exposures and confounders • larger number of controls enrolled to increase statistical power • multiple t-tests not performed to test numerous relationships • multivariate analyses used to assess independent effects raises many hypotheses about causes of newborn encephalopathy
Limitations	• causation between risk factors and newborn encephalopathy could not be inferred because of the chosen study design information of a small number of risk factors based on retrospective data may be biased by different recall of antepartum and intrapartum events in cases and controls

Matched case-control studies

In matched case-control studies, each of the control subjects is selected on the basis that they have characteristics, such as a certain age or gender, that match them with one of the study subjects. The design of a matched case-control study is shown in Figure 2.7.

Figure 2.7   Matched case-control study design

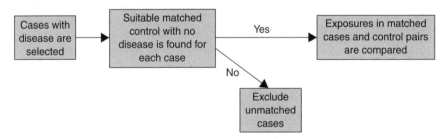

Matching is useful because it achieves a balance of important prognostic factors between the groups that may not occur by chance when random selection of controls is used, especially in small studies. Also, by effectively removing the effects of major confounders in the study design, it becomes easier to measure the true effect of the exposure under investigation. The underlying assumption is that if cases and controls are similar in terms of important confounders, then their differences can be attributed to a different exposure factor. An example of a typical matched case-control study is shown in Example 2.9.

Example 2.9 Matched case-control study Salonen et al. Relation between iron stores and non-insulin dependent diabetes in men: case-control study[44]	
Characteristic	**Description**
Aim	To measure the relationship between iron stores and non-insulin dependent diabetes
Type of study	Matched case-control study
Sample base	Random cross-sectional sample of 1038 men age 42–60
Follow-up period	4 years
Subjects	Cases: 41 men who developed non-insulin dependent diabetes during the follow-up period Controls: 82 diabetes-free subjects selected from sample base
Matching factors	Age, year, month of examination, place of residence, number of cigarettes smoked daily, exercise taken, maximal oxygen uptake, socioeconomic status, height, weight, hip and waist circumference and other serum vitamin and fatty acids
Outcome measurement	Diabetes defined as abnormal blood glucose level or receiving treatment for diabetes
Explanatory measurement	High iron store defined as ratio of concentration of ferritin receptors to ferritin in frozen serum samples in top quartile of sample
Statistics	Odds ratios
Conclusion	Men in the top quarter of the range of iron scores were at increased risk of developing diabetes (OR=2.4, 95% CI 1.0,5.5, P=0.04)
Strengths	• cases were drawn from a large random population sample • controls were selected from the same population • statistical power was increased by enrolling 2 controls for each case • objective measurements were used for defining the outcome and explanatory variables
Limitations	• the response rate at enrolment and the follow-up rate at 4 years are not reported so the effects of selection bias cannot be judged • controls are almost certainly over-matched, which may have reduced the estimate of effect • because of over-matching, the effects of other confounders in this study cannot be estimated • it is unclear whether an appropriate matched data analysis was used

Variables that are used for matching are often factors such as age, gender and ethnicity because these are strong confounders for many disease conditions. To match for these confounders, cases are often asked to nominate siblings or friends as controls. However, this type of matched control may also be more similar to the cases in regard to the exposure of interest. More appropriate controls are those that are matched by other population characteristics, such as by selecting the next live birth from a hospital at which a case is identified or by identifying the next person on the electoral register. The strengths and limitations of using matched controls are summarised in Table 2.7.

Table 2.7   Strengths and limitations of matched case-control studies

Strengths
- matching is an efficient method of controlling for major confounders
- matching for one factor (e.g. sibling) may also match for a range of other confounders such as ethnicity or socioeconomic status which may not be easy to measure
- selecting friends or family members increases the feasibility of recruiting control subjects

Limitations
- the effects of confounders that are used as matching variables cannot be investigated in the analyses
- selection bias occurs when cases are more likely to nominate friends who have similar exposures
- generalisability is reduced when the control group is more similar to the cases than to the general population
- controls need to be recruited after the cases are enrolled
- some cases may have to be excluded if a suitable control cannot be found
- analyses are limited to matched analyses in which only the exposures or characteristics of the discordant pairs are of interest
- the effective sample size is the number of pairs of subjects, not the total number of subjects in the study

---

In practice, matching is most useful for testing the effects of variables that are strongly related to both the exposure and to the outcome measurement with at least a four- or five-fold increase in risk. Matching does not provide an advantage in situations where the relation between the confounders and the exposure and outcome measurements is relatively weak. A disadvantage is that when friends or family members are recruited as matched controls, the exposures of the controls may not be independent of those of the cases. In this situation, the selection bias in the controls, because their exposures are not independent, can distort the odds ratio of effect by as much as two-fold magnitude in either direction, depending on the size and the direction of the bias.[45]

It is also important to avoid *over-matching*, which can be counterproductive[46] and which usually biases the results towards the null. The effects of this bias cannot be adjusted in the analyses. The concept of over-matching includes matching on too many confounders, on variables that are not confounders, or on inappropriate variables such as factors that are on the intermediate causal pathway between the disease and exposure under investigation. An example of over-matching is a study in which controls are matched to the cases on age, gender, ethnicity, occupation and socioeconomic status. In this type of study, the effects of smoking history would be expected to have a close association with both occupation and socioeconomic status and, as a result, the measured association between smoking history and the disease being investigated would be underestimated.

Despite the disadvantages, matching is a more efficient method with which to adjust for the effects of confounding than the use of multivariate statistical analyses.[47] However, the increase in precision that is achieved by matching is usually modest, that is a less than 20 per cent reduction in variance compared with the estimate obtained from multivariate analyses. In addition, matching on a factor that is strongly associated with the disease but not the exposure, or that is strongly associated with the exposure but not the disease, will give the correct estimate of effect but is likely to decrease precision. The advantages of matching also need to be balanced with the feasibility of recruiting the controls—in practice, if a match cannot be found then the case has to be excluded from the analyses, which leads to a loss of efficiency and generalisability.

Studies with historical controls

A study with a historical control group is one that compares a group of subjects who are all given the new treatment with a group of subjects who have all received the standard current treatment at some time in the past. An example of an intervention study with a historical control group is shown in Example 2.10.

Historical controls are usually used for convenience. The results from these types of studies will always be subject to bias because no blinding can be put in place and there are no methods that can be used to control for the effects of potential confounders. In such studies, no adjustment can be made for unpredicted differences between study groups such as subject characteristics that have not been measured, changes in inclusion criteria for other treatments, changes in methods used to measure exposure and outcome variables, or available treatments that change over time.

Example 2.10   Intervention study with a historical control group
Halken et al. Effect of an allergy prevention program on incidence of atopic symptoms in infancy[48]

Characteristic	Description
Aims	To investigate the effectiveness of allergen avoidance in the primary prevention of allergic symptoms in infancy
Type of study	Population based case-control study with historical controls
Sample base	'High-risk' infants, that is infants with high cord IgE and/or bi-parental atopic symptoms, born in specified region of Denmark
Subjects	Intervention group = 105 'high-risk' infants born in 1988 Controls = 54 'high-risk' infants born in 1985
Intervention	Avoidance of exposure to environmental tobacco smoke, pets and dust-collecting materials in the bedroom in the first 6 months of life
Follow-up period	Infants followed until age 18 months
Outcome measurements	Symptoms of recurrent wheeze, atopic dermatitis, etc. measured
Statistics	Chi-square tests used to determine differences in prevalence of symptoms between cases and controls
Conclusion	Allergen avoidance until the age of 6 months reduced the prevalence of recurrent wheeze during the first 18 months of life from 37% to 13% ($P < 0.01$)
Strengths	• first study to test the effectiveness of allergen avoidance as a primary preventive measure • birth cohort enrolled and intervention begun at earliest stage • results encourage the need for more rigorous trials
Limitations	• intervention not continued throughout trial • mixed intervention used so that the potentially effective or non-effective components are not known • no allergen exposure measurements collected • no measures used to reduce bias (randomisation, blinding etc.) • effects could be explained by factors other than the intervention (treatment, awareness, changed diet or use of childcare etc.)

Cross-sectional studies

In cross-sectional studies, a large random selection of subjects who are representative of a defined general population are enrolled and their health status, exposures, health-related behaviour, demographics and other relevant information are measured. As such, cross-sectional studies provide a useful 'snap-shot' of what is happening in a single study sample at one point in time.

Because both the exposures of interest and the disease outcomes are measured at the same time, no inference of which came first can be made. However, cross-sectional studies are ideal for collecting initial information about ideas of association, or for making an initial investigation into hypotheses about causal pathways. The design of a cross-sectional study is shown in Figure 2.8.

Figure 2.8   Design of a cross-sectional study

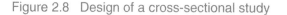

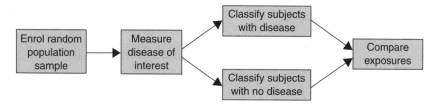

Glossary

Term	Meaning
Point prevalence	Number of cases of disease in a population within a specified time period
Cumulative prevalence	Total number of cases in the population who have ever had the disease
Incidence	Rate at which new cases of disease occur in a population
Mortality rate	Proportion of population that dies in a specified period

Cross-sectional studies are used to measure 'point' or 'cumulative' prevalence rates, associations between outcome and exposure measurements, or the effects of risk factors associated with a disease. The most appropriate use of cross-sectional studies is to collect information about the burden of disease in a community, either in terms of its prevalence, morbidity or mortality rates. In addition, serial cross-sectional studies are often used as a cheaper alternative to cohort studies for measuring trends in the changes of health status in a population, usually in chronic diseases such as diabetes, asthma or heart disease, or in health-related behaviours such as smoking. An example of a cross-sectional study is shown in Example 2.11.

Cross-sectional studies are an inexpensive first step in the process of identifying health problems and collecting information of possible risk factors. In cross-sectional studies, exposure and disease status is often collected by questionnaires that ask for current or retrospective information. To obtain a precise estimate of prevalence, a high response rate of over 80 per cent needs to be achieved in order to minimise the effects of selection bias.[49] Results from studies with a small sample size but with a high response rate are preferable to studies with a large sample but a low response rate because the generalisability of the results will be maximised. The features of study design that lead to bias in cross-sectional studies are shown in Table 2.8.

Table 2.8 Major sources of bias that influence estimates of prevalence and association in cross-sectional studies

Subjects
- non-random selection or a low response rate can lead to selection bias
- recall and reporting bias can influence the information collected

Measurements
- precision is reduced by large measurement error or poor validity of the methods
- may be influenced by observer bias

Example 2.11 Cross-sectional study
Kaur et al. Prevalence of asthma symptoms, diagnosis, and treatment in 12–14 year old children across Great Britain (ISAAC)[50]

Characteristic	Description
Aims	To measure variations in the prevalence of asthma symptoms in 12–14 year old children living in the UK
Type of study	Cross-sectional study
Sample base	All pupils in years with mostly 13–14 year-olds in selected state schools in specific regions in England, Wales and Scotland

Cont'd

Example 2.11 Cont'd   Cross-sectional study

Characteristic	Description
Sampling criteria	Schools randomly selected from prepared sampling frames
Subjects	27 507 children age 12–14 years enrolled of whom 49.2% were male; response rate was 86%
Outcome measurements	Symptoms and medication use collected by standardised questionnaire
Explanatory measurements	Regions throughout the world where similar studies conducted
Statistics	Prevalence rates
Conclusion	• 33% of children had wheezed in the last 12 months, 21% had a diagnosis of asthma and 16% used an asthma medication • these levels are higher than in previous studies or in studies of younger age groups and are amongst the highest in the world
Strengths	• schools were chosen randomly • methods were standardised between centres • a high response rate was achieved to minimise selection bias
Limitations	• only subjective outcome measurements collected • estimates of the presence of asthma may be influenced by reporting bias due to awareness, mis-diagnosis etc. • results apply only to these centres at the one point in time • no information of possible risk factors for asthma was collected

Ecological studies

In ecological studies, the units of observation are summary statistics from a population rather than measurements from individual subjects. Thus, the units of disease status may be assessed by incidence, prevalence or mortality rates from a population group such as a school, a geographic region, or a country, rather than from a sample of individual subjects. In addition, information on exposures is collected by proxy measurements such as information on socioeconomic status from a national census or regional humidity levels from a national bureau. An example of an ecological study is shown in Example 2.12.

Ecological studies are useful for describing variations between populations. As such, they can be used to assess whether an outcome of interest is different between groups rather than between individuals. A major limitation of ecological studies is that they provide a very weak study design for inferring causation because it is impossible to control for confounders. Also, associations may be difficult to detect if an unknown lag time occurs between secular trends in disease rates and in exposures to any explanatory risk factors.[51]

Example 2.12 Ecological study of SIDS mortality Douglas et al. Seasonality of sudden infant death syndrome in mainland Britain and Ireland 1985–1995.[52]	
Characteristic	Description
Aim	To examine whether sudden infant death syndrome (SIDS) occurs with a seasonal pattern
Type of study	Ecological
Outcome variable	SIDS death occurrences as documented by national database records
Explanatory variables	Season, year, age of child
Statistics	Effect of year and age on trends (curve fitting)
Conclusions	SIDS deaths occur with a seasonal peak in winter, especially in children aged less than 5 months old
Strengths	• informative collation and reporting of national data • useful background information for designing studies to measure risk factors
Limitations	• the accuracy of case ascertainment and its relation to other seasonally occurring illnesses is not known • there is no biological plausibility for the effect of season per se • no information was gained about the many possible confounders associated with season

Qualitative studies

Although this book is largely concerned with quantitative research, a description of qualitative studies is included for completeness. Qualitative studies are descriptive studies that use in-depth interviews to collect information. The characteristics of qualitative studies are described in Table 2.9. These types of studies are particularly useful for collecting information about the attitudes, perceptions or opinions of the subjects. As such, the content is dictated by the subject rather than by the measurement tools chosen by the researcher.

Table 2.9   Characteristics of qualitative studies
• they are an investigation of meaning and processes
• ask opinions rather than ranking feelings on a scale
• study behaviour from the subjects' perspectives
• lead to a better understanding of how the subjects think, feel or act
• can complement quantitative studies
• can identify broad questions that may be refined as the study progresses
• should aim, as far as possible, to study the subjects in their own environment
• can be used to formulate hypotheses or answer questions in their own right

Qualitative studies document behaviour and experience from the perspective of the patient or carer. As a result, qualitative studies are invaluable for collecting information about questions such as why some patients do not adhere to treatments, what patients require from their local health care systems, or what patients feel about changes in their health care. An example of a qualitative study is shown in Example 2.13.

Qualitative studies provide important information both in their own right[54, 55] and as an adjunct to quantitative studies.[56] In studies of effectiveness, it is often useful to collect qualitative data to explore the acceptability of the new treatment or intervention in addition to quantitative information to assess benefit. If an intervention proves to be ineffective, only qualitative data will provide information of whether the procedure or its side effects was unacceptable, or whether the treatment or intervention was too impractical to incorporate into daily routines. The value of collecting this type of information is shown in Example 2.14.

Example 2.13   Qualitative study
Butler et al. Qualitative study of patients' perceptions of doctors' advice
to quit smoking: implications for opportunistic health promotion[53]

Characteristic	Description
Aims	To assess the effectiveness and acceptability of opportunistic anti-smoking interventions conducted by general practitioners

Characteristic	Description
Type of study	Qualitative
Subjects	42 subjects in a smoking intervention program
Methods	Semi-structured interviews
Outcome measurements	Information about attempts to quit, thoughts on future smoking, past experiences with health services, and most appropriate way for health services to help them
Data analyses	Considered reduction of information into themes
Conclusions	Smokers • made their own evaluations about smoking • did not believe doctors could influence their smoking • believed that quitting was up to the individual • anticipated anti-smoking advice from their doctors, which made them feel guilty or annoyed
Implications	• a more informed approach to smoking cessation is needed • different approaches to smoking cessation by GPs may lead to better doctor–patient relationships for smokers
Strengths	• the information collected was much broader than could be obtained using a structured questionnaire • explanations for the failure of anti-smoking campaigns carried out by GPs can be used to further develop effective interventions
Limitations	• the generalisability of the results is not known

---

Example 2.14   Use of qualitative data to extend the information gained from a quantitative clinical trial

The effectiveness of a diet supplement in improving social function in girls with a congenital disorder was investigated in the blinded, placebo-controlled cross-over trial shown in Example 2.5. Analysis of the qualitative outcome measurements on a 5-point Likert scale suggested that the girls' functional abilities did not improve significantly during the active arm of the trial. However, qualitative data collected at semi-structured interviews showed that more than 70% of the parents or carers were able to judge when the subject was receiving the active treatment because of marked improvements in some specific functional abilities. In this study, the quantitative scales were not sensitive enough to detect improvements that were subtle but nevertheless of particular importance to parents and carers. If qualitative data had not been collected the treatment would have been judged to be ineffective, even though it resulted in substantial benefits for some patients and their carers.

Case reports or case series

Case reports or case series are a record of interesting medical cases. Case reports present a detailed medical history of the clinical and laboratory results for one patient or a small number of patients, whereas case series are descriptions of the medical history of larger numbers of patients.[57] These studies are entirely descriptive in that a hypothesis cannot be tested and associations cannot be explored by comparing the findings with another group of cases.

In both case reports and case series, the pattern of treatment and response is reported from a limited number of individual cases. An example of a case study is shown in Example 2.15.

Example 2.15   Case report of an unusual metabolic disorder
Ellaway et al. The association of protein-losing enteropathy with cobalamin C defect[58]

Characteristic	Description
Aim	To document a previously unreported association between protein-losing enteropathy and cobalamin C metabolic disorder
Type of study	Descriptive case report

Cont'd

Example 2.15 Cont'd   Case report on an unusual metabolic disorder

Characteristic	Description
Patient	Male infant of first cousin parents with birthweight below 10th percentile, poor feeding ability, failure to thrive and hospitalised for vomiting, diarrhoea and lethargy at age 4 weeks
Outcomes	Signs and symptoms; various haematological and biochemical tests
Statistics	None
Importance	Association not previously documented
Conclusion	• That physicians should consider this metabolic disorder in infants who fail to regain their birth weight
Strengths	• educational
Limitations	• the frequency and strength of the association is not known

Pilot studies and preliminary investigations

Pilot studies, which are sometimes called *feasibility studies*, are necessary to ensure that practical problems in the study protocol are identified. This ensures that the protocol does not need to be changed once the planned study is underway and therefore, that standardised, high quality data will be collected. The uses of pilot studies are shown in Table 2.10. An essential feature of a pilot study is that the data are not used to test a hypothesis or included with data from the actual study when the results are reported.

Table 2.10   Processes that can be evaluated in pilot studies
• the quality of the data collection forms and the accuracy of the instruments
• the practicalities of conducting the study
• the success of recruitment approaches
• the feasibility of subject compliance with tests
• estimates for use in sample size calculations

The uses of *internal pilot studies*, in which the data are part of the data set that is used to test the study hypothesis on completion of the study, are discussed in Chapter 4.

Occasionally, studies with a small sample size are conducted to evaluate whether a larger, more definitive study to test a hypothesis is warranted. These studies are not pilot studies in the classical sense described in

Table 2.10 and, to avoid confusion, are probably best described as a *preliminary investigation*. Because such studies should always be capable of answering a research question in their own right, the study design and subject selection should be appropriate and the sample size should be adequate.

Strengths and limitations of study designs

Each type of study design has its own inherent strengths and limitations. However, all studies have their place in the larger scheme of collecting data that is sufficiently convincing for a new treatment or health care practice to be introduced, for a new method to replace previous methods, or for a public health intervention to be implemented. The inherent strengths and limitations of each of the types of study design that have been described are summarised in Table 2.11.

In epidemiological research, associations between exposures and diseases are usually investigated in a progressive way in order to avoid wasting valuable research resources. In many situations, it is pragmatic to tread a conservative path and first assess whether a relation exists in cheaper studies that provide more rapid answers, such as ecological, cross-sectional or case-control studies. If a study of this type confirms that a significant association is likely to exist, then it is reasonable to progress to a more definitive study. This may involve undertaking a cohort study or non-randomised trial before finally conducting a randomised controlled trial to test the effects of intervening, if this is feasible and appropriate.

It is also important to tread a considered path that conserves research resources when planning a clinical study to test the effects of new treatments or interventions on morbidity due to ill health. For this reason, evidence of new treatment modalities is usually first collected in preliminary investigations such as Phase I studies, or by using a cheaper study design such as a case-control study before more definitive evidence of efficacy, effectiveness or equivalence is collected in various forms of randomised controlled trials.

Table 2.11 Strengths and limitations of study design		
Type of study	Strengths	Limitations
Systematic review	• summarises current information • directs need for new studies	• bias can occur if methods for each study are not standardised and some studies have a small sample size

Cont'd

Table 2.11 Cont'd   Strengths and limitations of study design

Type of study	Strengths	Limitations
Randomised controlled trials	• scientifically rigorous • provide the most convincing evidence • control for known and unknown confounders	• expensive and difficult to conduct • generalisability may be poor • may not be ethically feasible
Cohort studies	• can document progression of disease • reduce effects of recall bias • can be used to measure incidence rates • provide information of the timing of events and risk factors	• expensive to conduct • prevention of loss to follow-up may be impossible • require large sample size especially for studies of rare diseases • exposure may be linked to unknown confounders • blinding is not always possible
Non-randomised clinical trials	• can answer important clinical questions	• evidence is only supplemental to randomised controlled trials
Case-control studies	• easy to conduct and provide rapid results • large sample size not required • suitable for study of rare diseases • important first stage in investigating risk factors	• difficult to control for bias and confounding • may be difficult to recruit suitable controls • information about exposure relies on subject recall
Cross-sectional studies	• fast and easy to conduct • can provide accurate estimates of prevalence • provide initial information of associations and risk factors	• random sample may be difficult to recruit • prone to bias if response rate low • effect of timing of exposure cannot be estimated
Ecological studies	• quick and easy • can generate hypotheses	• not possible to control for confounders • time lags may influence results

Cont'd

Table 2.11 Cont'd   Strengths and limitations of study design

Type of study	Strengths	Limitations
Qualitative studies	• provide information from a patient perspective	• cannot be used to test a hypothesis
Case reports or case series	• provide new information	• cannot be used to test a hypothesis
Preliminary investigations	• help decide whether a study is warranted	• need to be followed by a more definitive study
Pilot studies	• ensure quality data	• cannot be used to test a hypothesis

Methodological studies

In research studies, the extent to which measurements are accurate (repeatable) or to which one instrument can be used interchangeably with another instrument (agreement) are fundamental issues that influence the study results. Because of this, it is important that these issues are established before data collection begins. To conserve accuracy, studies in which the repeatability or agreement is being evaluated must be designed so that they do not produce a falsely optimistic or a falsely pessimistic impression of the accuracy of the instrument. The important issues when designing a study to estimate repeatability or agreement are shown in Table 2.12.

Table 2.12   Study design for measuring repeatability or agreement

- the conditions under which measurements are taken are identical on each occasion
- the equipment is identical and the same protocol is followed on each occasion
- at subsequent tests, both subject and observer are blinded to the results of the prior tests
- each subject must have exactly the same number of observations
- subjects are selected to represent the entire range of measurements that can be encountered
- no new treatment or clinical intervention is introduced in the period between measurements
- the time between measurements is short enough so that the severity of the condition being measured has not changed
- a high follow-up rate is attained

Section 2—Random error and bias

The objectives of this section are to understand:
- how bias can arise in a research study;
- how to minimise bias in the study design; and
- how to assess the influence of bias.

Measuring associations

Most clinical and epidemiological research studies are designed to measure associations between an exposure and the presence of a disease, which may be measured as improvement, prevention or worsening of symptoms. An exposure can be an environmental factor, a treatment or an intervention. Figure 2.9 shows how the strength of the association that is measured in any type of study can be significantly influenced by factors that are a direct result of the study design and the methods used. This section discusses how random error and bias can arise, and can be prevented, in order to make an estimate of association that is closer to the truth.

Figure 2.9   Factors that influence associations

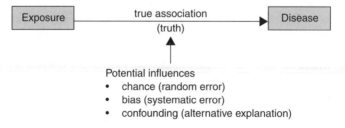

Bias

Bias is the difference between the study results and the truth. As such, bias is a major problem that has to be considered in the design of research studies because it is not possible to adjust for the effects of bias at a later stage, such as in the data analyses. Thus, the research studies that are designed to have the least potential for bias are the studies that have the most potential to produce reliable results. Because systematic bias distorts the study results and because the magnitude and direction can be difficult to predict, detection and avoidance are fundamental considerations in all research studies.

Bias is not related to sample size. The effects of bias on the study results remain the same whatever the sample size, so that a large study that has a significant bias is no better than a small study with a significant bias – it only serves to waste more resources. The only satisfactory methods for minimising the potential for bias are to design studies carefully to ensure that the sampling procedures are reliable and to implement all procedures using standardised methods to ensure that the measurements are accurate when the data are collected.

Random error

Random error is sometimes called *non-systematic bias*. Most measurements have some degree of random error but, because this occurs to a similar extent in all subjects regardless of study group, it is less of a problem than non-random error, or *systematic bias*. Measurements that are more susceptible to interpretation and that therefore have a low degree of repeatability, such as a tape measure for estimating height, will have far more random error than an item of calibrated equipment such as a stadiometer, which provides much better precision by reducing random error. In clinical and epidemiological studies, misclassification errors in assigning subjects to the correct disease or exposure groups can also cause random error.

Random error always results in a bias towards the null, that is a bias towards a finding of no association between two variables. Thus, the effects of random error are more predictable, and therefore less serious, than the effects of systematic bias. In Figure 2.10, the solid curves show the frequency distribution of a continuous measurement taken from two groups, A and B. If random error is present, the 'noise' around the measurements is greater and the distributions will be broader as shown by the dotted curves. Because this type of error always tends to make the study groups more alike by increasing the amount of overlap in their distributions, it will lead to an increase in the standard deviation of the measurement, and therefore to under-estimation of effect.

Figure 2.10   Effect of random error

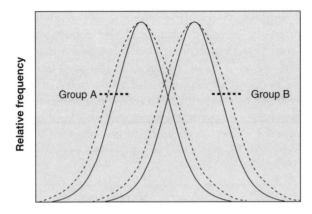

The solid lines show the frequency distribution of a measurement in two study groups, A and B. The dotted lines show how the frequency of the same measurement would be distributed if there was additional random error around the estimates.

Systematic bias

Systematic bias, which is often called *differential bias* or *non-random error*, is the most serious type of bias because it leads to an under-estimation or an over-estimation of results, or to an incorrect statistically significant or insignificant difference between study groups. In many situations, systematic bias has an unpredictable effect so that the direction of the bias on the results is difficult to detect. The types of bias that are likely to lead to an over-estimation or under-estimation of effect are shown in Figure 2.11.

Figure 2.11   Effects of systematic bias

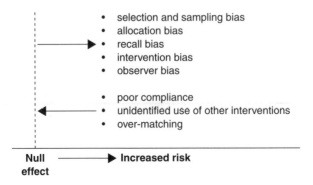

Systematic bias often occurs when the response rate in a study is low or when the study methods or sampling criteria create an artificial differ-ence in the association between the exposure and the outcome in the cases and controls, or in the sampled group and the population. The effect of systematic bias may be to either increase or decrease a measured incidence or prevalence rate, or to increase or decrease the association between two variables, such as between an exposure and an outcome or between a treat-ment and the severity of symptoms. An over-estimation of association can occur if the assessment of outcome becomes biased because an association is thought to exist by either the subject or the observer.[59]

Glossary

Term	Meaning
Under-estimation	Finding of a weaker association between two variables or a lower prevalence rate than actually exists
Over-estimation	Finding of a stronger association between two variables or a higher prevalence rate than actually exists
Misclassification of subjects	Classification of cases as controls, or vice-versa
Misclassification of exposure	Classification of exposed subjects as non-exposed, or vice-versa

Some common sources of systematic bias are shown in Table 2.13, and an example of the effect of systematic recall bias is shown in Example 2.16. The association shown in the study outlined in Example 2.16 would be rendered non-significant by a very modest degree of recall bias.[60]

Table 2.13   Sources of systematic bias

Subjects
- have an interest in the relationship being investigated
- have different exposures or outcomes to non-responders
- selectively recall or over-report exposures that are not a personal choice, such as occupational or industrial exposures
- selectively under-report exposures that are a personal choice, such as smoking or alcohol use

Researchers
- have an interest in the relationship being investigated
- are not blinded to study group
- estimate the exposure or outcome differently in the cases and controls

Example 2.16 Study with potential systematic recall bias Fontham et al. Environmental tobacco smoke and lung cancer in non-smoking women[61]	
Characteristic	Description
Aims	To measure the risk of lung cancer in lifetime non-smokers exposed to environmental tobacco smoke
Type of study	Population based case-control study
Sample base	Female lifetime non-smokers in five metropolitan centres in the USA
Subjects	653 cases with confirmed lung cancer and 1253 controls selected by random digit dialing and random sampling from health registers
Outcome measurements	Lung cancer confirmed with histology
Exposure measurements	In-person interviews to measure retrospective reporting of tobacco use and exposure to environmental tobacco smoke (proxy reporting by next of kin for sick or deceased cases); tobacco smoke exposure from mother, father, spouse or other household members measured
Statistics	Logistic regression to estimate odds ratios adjusted for confounders, e.g. age, race, study centre, anti-oxidant intake
Conclusion	exposure to smoking by a spouse increases the risk of lung cancer in lifetime non-smokers with an odds ratio of approximately 1.3 (P<0.05)
Strengths	• large sample size allowed effect to be measured with precision, i.e. with small confidence interval • disease status of cases confirmed with diagnostic tests i.e. misclassification bias of cases is minimised • controls sampled randomly from population i.e. selection bias is minimised • demographic characteristics well balanced in case and control groups i.e. effects of confounders minimised
Limitations	• information bias likely to be high in 37% of cases for whom proxy measurements had to be collected • likely to be significant systematic recall of tobacco and diet exposures between cases and controls • the odds ratios of effect are small so that only a modest degree of systematic recall bias may explain the result[62]

Types of bias

Bias can arise from three sources: the subjects, the researchers or the measurements used. The terms that are used to describe specific sources of bias are listed in Table 2.14. The studies that are most prone to measurement bias, because they often rely on retrospective reporting by the subjects who are aware of their disease classification, are case-control and cross-sectional studies. Cohort studies in which exposures and symptom history are measured prospectively rather than relying on recall tend to be less prone to some biases.

Table 2.14 Types of bias that can occur in research studies	
Bias	Alternative terms and subsets
Selection bias	Sampling bias Non-response bias Volunteer or self-selection bias Allocation bias Follow-up or withdrawal bias Ascertainment bias
Intervention bias	Bias due to poor compliance Different treatment of study groups
Measurement bias	Observer or recorder bias Information bias Misclassification bias Recall or reporting bias
Analysis and publication bias	Interpretation bias Assumption bias

Selection bias

Selection bias, which is sometimes called *sampling* bias, is a systematic difference in terms of exposures or outcomes between subjects enrolled for study and those not enrolled. This leads to an under-estimation or over-estimation of descriptive statistics, such as prevalence rates, or of association statistics, such as odds ratios. When subjects are selected using non-random methods or when subjects self-select themselves into groups, there is a large potential for selection bias to occur. There is also potential for selection bias between patients who consent to enrol in a clinical study or in a population study and those who choose not to participate.

A major effect of selection bias is that it reduces the external validity of the study; that is, the generalisability of the results to the community. For this reason, it is important to use careful sampling procedures and to adhere strictly to any inclusion and exclusion criteria so that the characteristics of the study sample can be described precisely and the generalisability of the results can be accurately described.

Glossary

Term	Meaning
Generalisability	Extent to which the study results can be applied to the target population
Confounders	Factors that are associated with the outcome and the exposure being studied but are not part of the causal pathway
Prognostic factors	Factors that predict a favourable or unfavourable outcome

In cross-sectional studies, a major source of selection bias is *non-response bias*. Non-response bias causes an under-estimation or an over-estimation of prevalence rates if a non-representative sample is enrolled. Because the amount of bias may increase as the response rate decreases, a minimum response rate of 80 per cent is thought necessary for cross-sectional studies from which prevalence rates are being reported, and response rates below 60 per cent are thought to be inadequate.[63]

The situations in which selection bias can occur in non-randomised clinical trials, cohort studies and case-control studies are shown in Table 2.15. The many sources of bias that can arise and the difficulties in controlling the bias preclude these types of studies from being useful for providing definitive evidence of causation between an exposure and a disease, or evidence of the effectiveness of a treatment.

Table 2.15   Situations in which selection bias may occur in non-random trials, and in cohort and cross-sectional studies

Subjects
- self-select themselves into a trial or a study
- have different characteristics that are related to outcome than the refusers
- are more educated or lead a healthier lifestyle than refusers
- have a better or worse prognosis than refusers

Researchers
- selectively allocate subjects to a treatment group
- use different selection criteria for the intervention and control groups, or the exposed and non-exposed groups
- are aware of the purpose of the study and of the subject's exposure to the factor of interest

In matched case-control studies, matching is used to control for factors, such as age or gender, that are important confounders in a relationship between an exposure and a disease. In these types of studies, it is often both convenient and cost effective to ask cases to nominate control subjects who are their friends or relatives. Selection bias is a significant problem when this type of selection process is used. The use of friends and relatives as controls can inadvertently result in 'over-matching' for the exposure of interest, which will bias the results towards the null.

Glossary

Term	Meaning
Inclusion criteria	Subject characteristics that determine inclusion in a study
Exclusion criteria	Subject characteristics that determine exclusion from being enrolled in a study
Response rate	Proportion of eligible subjects who are enrolled in a study
Compliance	Regularity with which subjects adhere to study protocol, e.g. take medications or record outcome measurements

A type of selection bias called *allocation bias* occurs when there is a difference in the characteristics of subjects who are allocated to the separate treatment groups in a clinical trial.[64, 65] Differential allocation may result in an imbalance in prognostic factors or confounders and can have a strong influence on the results. The effects of these types of allocation biases can be minimised by using efficient randomisation methods to allocate subjects to treatment or to control groups, and by blinding the observers to the allocation procedures.

Glossary

Term	Meaning
Exposure group	Group who have been exposed to the environmental factor being studied
Intervention group	Group receiving the new treatment being studied or undertaking a new environmental intervention
Placebo group	Group receiving a sham treatment that has no effect and is indistinguishable by subjects from the active treatment
Control group	Group with which the effect of the treatment or exposure of interest is compared

Follow-up bias is a major problem in cohort studies. This type of bias occurs when the subjects remaining in the study are systematically different from those who are lost to follow-up. Follow-up bias becomes a systematic bias when follow-up rates are related to either the measurements of exposure or to the outcome. For example, subjects who have a disease that is being studied may be more likely to stay in a study than healthy control subjects, who may be more likely to drop out. An example of a study in which there was a strong potential for follow-up bias is shown in Example 2.17.

Follow-up bias can also occur when subjects who suspect that their disease is related to a past occupational exposure may be more likely to remain in the study than control subjects who have no such suspicions. In clinical trials, follow-up bias has an important effect when cases drop out because of side effects due to the intervention, or because they recover earlier than the subjects in the control group. Estimates of effect can become distorted when the follow-up rate is different in the intervention and control groups. The only way to minimise this type of bias is to use multiple methods to maximise follow-up rates in all of the study groups.

Example 2.17 Study with potential for follow-up bias	
Peat et al. Serum IgE levels, atopy and asthma in young adults: results from a longitudinal cohort study[66]	
Characteristic	**Description**
Aims	To explore the natural history of asthma from childhood to early adulthood and its relation to allergic responses
Type of study	Longitudinal cohort study
Sample base	Population sample of 718 children studied at age 8–10 years
Subjects	180 subjects restudied at age 18–20 years
Outcome measurements	Asthmatic symptoms, airway hyper-responsiveness to histamine (AHR), skin prick tests and serum IgE
Statistics	Analysis of variance, trends and chi-square tests of association
Conclusion	• serum IgE and atopy have an important dose-response relation with AHR in young adults, even in the absence of asthmatic symptoms • subjects who had AHR or symptoms in early childhood had a high probability of very high serum IgE levels in later life

Cont'd

Example 2.17 Cont'd   Study with potential for follow-up bias

Characteristic	Description
Strengths	A lifelong history of asthma symptoms could be collected prospectively thereby reducing recall bias
Limitations	• only 57% of the original sample were enrolled in the follow-up study and less than half of these subjects agreed to have blood taken for serum IgE measurements (25% of original sample) • no inferences about the prevalence of any characteristics could be made • effects of follow-up bias unknown so that generalisability is unclear

Intervention bias

Intervention bias occurs when the intervention and control groups act, or are treated, differently from one another. Intervention bias may lead to an over-estimation of effect when there is a greater use of diagnostic or treatment procedures in the intervention group than in the control group, or when subjects in the intervention group are contacted or studied more frequently than those in the control group. Intervention bias can also lead to an under-estimation of effect between groups when there is an unidentified use of an intervention in the control group. To reduce intervention bias, it is important to standardise all of the treatment and data collection methods that are used.

An example of potential intervention bias was identified in a randomised controlled trial of the effects of the Buteyko method, which is an alternative breathing therapy for asthma.[67] The results from this study suggested that the Buteyko method significantly reduced the self-reported use of pharmacological medications and marginally improved quality of life in patients with asthma. However, the effect may have been over-estimated because the active intervention group was contacted by telephone much more frequently than the control group subjects. This failure to standardise the amount of contact with all study subjects could have influenced the self-reporting of outcomes by creating a greater expectation of benefit in the active treatment group.[68] When designing a study, it is important to anticipate these types of bias so that their effects can be minimised when conducting the study.

Poor compliance in the intervention group can also bias results towards the null by leading to an inaccurate estimation of the dose required to achieve a specific effect. If 25 per cent of subjects are non-compliant, the sample size will need to be increased by up to 50 per cent in order to maintain the statistical power to demonstrate an effect. Common methods that are used to improve compliance include the use of written instructions, frequent reminders, and providing supplies. Any methods that improve compliance will have the potential to lead to more accurate estimates of the true effects of new treatments or interventions. However, the methods used become an integral part of the intervention.

Measurement bias

Measurement bias, which is sometimes called *information bias*, occurs when the outcome or the exposure is misclassified. The situations in which measurement bias commonly occur are shown in Table 2.16. Solutions to avoid measurement bias include the use of measurements that are as accurate as possible, ensuring that both the observers and the subjects are blinded to study group status, and employing objective measurements wherever possible.[69]

The term *measurement bias* is usually used if the measurement is continuous, or *misclassification bias* if the measurement is categorical. A situation in which measurement bias can occur is when heart rate is documented when the subject is nervous or has been hurrying rather than when the subject is calm and sedentary. Because of the potential for measurement bias to occur, it is important to ensure that all measurements are collected using standardised methods so that both observer and subject biases are minimised. An example of a study that was designed to measure the extent to which systematic misclassification bias was present is shown in Example 2.18. Although misclassification bias affects the classification of exposures and outcomes in almost all studies, its effects cannot usually be quantified unless an appropriate validation study has been conducted.

Table 2.16   Sources of measurement bias

Subjects
- selectively under-report or over-report exposure to lifestyle choices such as dietary intakes, cigarette smoking, or alcohol intake
- do not answer sensitive questions, such as income, accurately
- selectively recall events once the disease of interest occurs

Researchers
- are aware of group status

Measurements
- conditions under which measurements are taken are not standardised
- questionnaires developed for one particular age group or clinical setting are used in a different setting

---

Observer bias may occur when the subject or the investigator is aware of the group to which the subject has been allocated or the status of the exposure being investigated. It is important to minimise observer bias by using objective outcome measurements[70] or by having carefully trained investigators with efficient blinding procedures in place.[71] Observer bias can also be minimised by using more than one source of information, for example by verifying the outcomes or exposures with information available from external sources such as medical or vaccination records.

Another type of measurement bias is *recall bias*. This type of bias can occur in case-control and cross-sectional studies in which retrospective data are collected from the subjects. Recall bias arises when there are differences in the memory of significant past exposures between cases and controls. For example, parents of children with a neurodevelopment disorder, such as cerebral palsy, often have a much sharper recall of exposures and events that occurred during pregnancy or during delivery than the parents of healthy children.

Reporting bias may lead to over- or under-estimates of prevalence rates. This commonly occurs in situations in which subjects report information about other members of their family, such as parents reporting on behalf of their children. For example, parents may under-report symptoms of wheeze following exercise in their child if they are not always present when their child has been exercising. Another example of reporting bias is proxy reports by women of the number of cigarettes or amount of alcohol consumed by their partners. In a study of pregnant women, approximately 30 per cent of replies between women and their partners were not in agreement.[72] Reporting bias may also distort measures of association when subjects selectively report or withhold information. For example, a systematic under-reporting of smoking in pregnancy will tend to underestimate the association between maternal smoking and low birth weight because some smokers will be classified as non-smokers.

Analysis and publication bias

Bias can also arise during data analysis when data are 'dredged' before a positive result is found, when interim analyses are repeatedly undertaken as the study progresses, or when problem cases (such as those with exclusion criteria or with outlying or missing values) are mishandled. Analysis bias can also arise if 'intention-to-treat' analyses are not used when reporting the results from randomised controlled trials, when only selected subjects are included in the analysis, or when subjects are regrouped for analysis by their exposure status rather than by initial group allocation. These methods will tend to remove the balance of confounding that was achieved by randomising the subjects to groups.

Glossary

Term	Meaning
Categorical variable	Variable that can be divided into discrete categories, e.g. Yes/No or 1, 2, 3, 4
Continuous variable	Variable measured on a continuous scale, e.g. height or weight
Intention-to-treat analysis	Analysis with all subjects included in group to which they are originally randomised regardless of non-compliance, completion in trial etc.
Missing values	Data points that were not collected, e.g. due to non-attendance, inability to perform tests etc.
Interim analyses	Analyses conducted before entire subject enrolment is completed

Assumption bias may arise from mistaken interpretations of the association between variables as a result of illogical reasoning or inappropriate data analyses. Similarly, *interpretation bias* may arise from a restricted interpretation of the results that fails to take account of all prior knowledge.

Publication bias occurs because positive findings are more likely to be reported and published in the journals[73] or because covert duplicate publication of data can occur.[74] Publication bias may also arise as a result of hypotheses being based on a single piece of positive evidence rather than all of the evidence available, or as a result of authors omitting to discuss reservations about the conclusions. Other sources of publication bias include the delayed or failed publication of studies with negative results.

In systematic reviews, bias can be introduced in meta-analyses if the review is more likely to include positive trials, a large proportion of small trials that have greater random fluctuation in their estimates, or trials published in only one language.[75, 76] Results can also be biased if data from subgroups that are expected to respond differently are combined. In addition, results will be biased towards a more favourable outcome if fixed rather than random effects models are used to summarise the results when heterogeneity between studies is expected.[77]

Estimating the influence of bias

While it is impossible to adjust for bias in data analyses, it is sometimes possible to make an estimation of its effect on the results or on the conclusions of a study. The effect of selection bias can be estimated using *sensitivity analyses* if some information of non-responders has been collected.

Sensitivity analyses simply involves the recalculation of statistics such as the prevalence rate or odds ratio using one of the methods shown in Table 2.17. The application of a sensitivity analysis is shown in Example 2.18.

Table 2.17   Methods for sensitivity analyses
• assume that all, or a proportion of non-responders, do or do not have the disease of interest and then recalculate upper and lower bounds of prevalence • estimate the extent of misclassification, e.g. the proportion of non-smokers who are thought to be smokers, and then recalculate the odds ratio • exclude or include the expected proportion of inaccurate replies

In some situations, it is possible to collect data that can be used to assess the effect of any systematic bias on the results. For example, questionnaires may be used in a study in which it is not practical or economically feasible to measure true exposures in the entire sample. In this case, it is sometimes possible to collect accurate information of true exposures in a smaller study and use this to validate the questionnaire responses in order to ascertain whether there is any measurement bias.[78]

Example 2.18   Application of a sensitivity analysis

Say, for example, that a prevalence study of asthma in young children is conducted and the response rate is only 70%. If no information of non-responders can be obtained, a sensitivity analysis can be conducted to estimate the effect on prevalence if the rate of asthma in the non-responders was, say, half or double that in the responders. The calculations are as follows.
Total size of population = 1400 children
Number of children studied = 980 (response rate 70%)
Number of non-responders = 420 children
Number of children with asthma in study sample of 980 children = 186
Prevalence of children with asthma in study sample = 186 / 980 = 18.9%
Prevalence of children with asthma in population if rate in
     non-responders is 9.5% = (186 + 40) / 1400 = 16.1%
Prevalence of children with asthma in population if rate in
     non-responders is 38% = (186 + 160) / 1400 = 24.7%
The estimates in the non-responders and the effect they have on the estimation of prevalence are shown in Figure 2.12. The sensitivity analysis suggests that the true rate of asthma in the population is likely to be in the range of 16.1% to 24.7%. However, this estimate is not precise because it relies on a subjective judgment of the response rate in the non-responders.

Figure 2.12   Sensitivity analysis

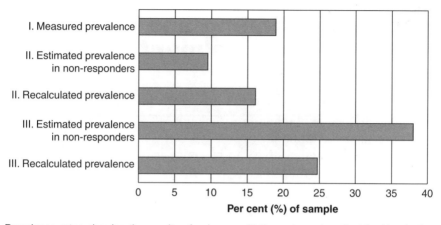

Prevalence rates showing the results of using sensitivity analyses to adjust for bias in the characteristics of non-responders in a study.

For cross-sectional studies, more complicated methods are available, including the use of sampling weights to adjust for the effects of greater non-response from some sections of a population. These methods can be used to adjust for systematic bias due to the effects of factors such as socioeconomic status on the response rate.[79]

For case-control studies, statistical methods have been developed to quantify the extent of systematic recall bias that would be required to overturn the results of the study.[80] Such analyses involve recalculating the odds ratio using estimations of the probability that an exposed subject has been recorded as being unexposed, or an unexposed subject has been recorded as being exposed. These probabilities can be estimated if prior studies to validate exposure measurements, such as measurements estimated by questionnaires, have been undertaken. By conducting such analyses, it is possible to determine the extent to which the conclusions remain valid under a range of systematic recall bias situations.

Section 3—Blinding and allocation concealment

The objectives of this section are to understand:
- the importance of blinding in reducing bias;
- how to implement blinding;
- why allocation methods have to be concealed; and
- the problems of conducting interim analyses.

Blinding is an essential tool for reducing bias in research studies. Studies are called 'single-blinded' when either the subjects or the observers are unaware of the group to which subjects have been allocated, or 'double-blinded' when both the subjects and the observers are unaware of group status. Subject blinding is a fundamental consideration in clinical trials, whereas observer blinding is a fundamental issue in all types of research studies.

Subject blinding

In clinical trials, subjects should be unaware of, that is blinded to, the group to which they have been allocated.[81] Blinding is sometimes achieved with the use of a placebo treatment, that is an inert substance that looks and tastes the same as the active treatment. Alternatively, in intervention studies, a sham intervention can be used in the control group. This is important in trials of new treatments or interventions in which a 'placebo effect' may occur, that is a situation in which patients perceive a psychological benefit from a treatment that is not related to the inherent efficacy of the treatment.

The direction of any 'placebo effect' can be difficult to judge because this may arise from the expectation that the new treatment will have a greater benefit, or the assurance that the standard treatment is more effective. It is not uncommon for patients who are involved in clinical trials to report a more optimistic account of their symptoms simply out of willingness to please the researchers who have been trying to help and who are interested in all aspects of their clinical outcomes.

In epidemiological studies in which questionnaires or subject interviews are used to collect outcome and exposure data, subjects should be unaware of the relationship that is being investigated. This is also important in case-control studies in which subjects are asked to recall exposures that happened at some time in the past.

Observer blinding

In all research studies, procedures need to be in place to ensure that observers or assessors are as objective as possible when assessing outcomes. In most studies, bias can be minimised by the assessors being unaware (blinded) to the group or exposure status of the subjects. Most clinical trials are designed with the expectation that there will be a difference between groups. However, the very expectation that the new or active treatment will be better or worse than the current or placebo treatment has the potential to lead to a difference in the conduct or frequency of follow-up procedures between the groups. These expectations may also lead to a more optimistic or pessimistic interpretation of the outcome measurements in the active or new treatment groups.

In epidemiological studies in which an association between an exposure and an outcome is being investigated, bias can be avoided by the researchers who are assessing outcomes being blinded to the subjects' exposure status, and by the researchers who are assessing the subjects' exposure status being blinded to subjects' outcome status.

Allocation concealment

In randomised and non-randomised trials, all correct guesses about group allocation by the researchers responsible for recruiting subjects have the potential to lead to allocation bias. Because of this, random allocation and allocation concealment are important tools that overcome any intentional or unintentional influences in the researcher who is responsible for allocating subjects to a trial group. With efficient allocation and concealment in place, the group allocation of the subjects should be determined entirely by chance.

Allocation concealment is important because some researchers indulge in ingenious efforts to decipher allocation codes. In studies in which the researchers who are responsible for enrolling the subjects are curious about group allocation and treat breaking the code as an intellectual challenge, only a strategic randomisation allocation plan and an efficient concealment policy can reduce bias.[82]

A basic requirement of allocation concealment is that researchers who prepare the random allocation scheme should not be involved in the recruitment processes or in assessing outcomes. Conversely, researchers who are recruiting subjects should not be involved in selecting and undertaking the random allocation procedure. Concealment is essential because it has been estimated that larger treatment effects are reported from trials with inadequate allocation concealment.[83] Because the methods of concealment are just as important as those of allocation, many journals now require that these methods are reported.

Many ways of concealing allocated codes can be used. In small trials, sealed envelopes are commonly used because of their simplicity, but lists held by a third person such as a pharmacy or central control by phone are the preferred method. Obviously, the sequence is more easily determined if the observers are not blinded to the treatment group but in studies in which effective double-blinding is in place, the use of a placebo that is as similar as possible to the active drug can help to maintain concealment. In this type of study, the preferred concealment method is the use of previously numbered or coded containers.

When minimisation methods are being used to randomise subjects to groups, it is especially important to conceal information of the predictive factors being used in the process and to conceal their distribution in the trial groups from the researchers who are responsible for recruiting the subjects.

Documentation

Although random allocation should follow a pre-determined plan, specifications of the precise methods are not usually included in the protocol or in other documentation because this would make them accessible to the staff responsible for data collection and would circumvent effective allocation concealment. However, once recruitment is complete, the method can be openly reported. When publishing the results of the trial, it is essential that both the methods of randomisation and of concealment are reported together.[84]

Methodological studies

Blinding is an important concept for reducing bias in methodological studies such as those designed to measure the repeatability of an instrument, the agreement between two different instruments or the diagnostic utility of a clinical tool. In these types of studies, it is important that the observers who make the measurements are blinded to the 'gold standard', to other measurements or to the results of prior diagnostic tests in each subject.[85] In such studies, blinding is the only method to ensure that expectation on the part of the observers does not make the instruments that will be used to assess clinical outcome measurements seem better or worse than they actually are.

Interim analyses

In all research studies but in clinical trials particularly, interim analyses should be planned before data collection begins. More importantly, the results of interim analyses that are undertaken before data collection is complete should not be available to the team who are continuing to collect the data. If the results become available, there may be an expectation on the part of the research team or the subjects that further data collection should follow a certain pattern. The expectation may be that further data will follow the direction of the interim results, or that larger differences will need to be found before a difference between groups becomes significant. These expectations have the potential to bias all data collection that follows the interim analysis.

In many large trials, bias is avoided by blinding the data management and data analysis teams to the coding of the 'group' variable in the database. In this way, expectations that the data should behave in one way or another are less likely to influence the final results.

Resources required

In any research study, efficient blinding practices require adequate resources in order to implement the procedures. To reduce bias, the people who are responsible for randomly allocating subjects to study groups should be different to the people responsible for collecting data, and both positions should be independent of the responsibility for maintaining the database and conducting the interim analyses. This requires a greater commitment of resources than in studies in which researchers are required to perform multiple roles, but is always worthwhile in terms of minimising bias.

3

CHOOSING THE MEASUREMENTS

Section 1—Outcome measurements

The objectives of this section are to understand:
- how to select appropriate outcome measurements;
- the relative benefits of objective and subjective measurements; and
- how to reduce measurement error in clinical trials.

Choice of outcome measurements

Much care is needed when choosing the outcome and explanatory variables that will be used to test the main hypotheses in a research study. Because no adjustment for unreliable or invalid measurements can be made in the analyses, it is important to use both outcome and explanatory measurements that are as precise and as valid as possible. This will improve the likelihood of being able to accurately measure the impact of interventions, or to measure the associations between two factors with accuracy. The essential features of accurate outcome measurements are shown in Table 3.1.

Table 3.1   Essential qualities of accurate measurements
• good face and content validity
• good criterion or construct validity
• repeatable
• good between-observer agreement
• responsive to change

Good face and content validity are both essential characteristics of outcome measurements because they ensure that the measurement identifies the symptoms and illnesses that are important in clinical terms and that are relevant to the aims of the study. In addition, measurements with good criterion or construct validity are valuable because they measure what they are expected to measure with as much accuracy as possible. It is also essential that measurements have good between-observer agreement and are precise, or repeatable. The issues of validity are described later in this chapter, and the methods that can be used to establish repeatability and agreement are described in Chapter 7.

Glossary

Term	Meaning
Subject error	Error caused by subject factors such as compliance with exertion when taking measurements of lung function, or recent exercise when taking measurements of blood pressure
Observer error	Variations in assessment due to differences between observers in the method used to administer a test or to interpret the result
Instrument error	Changes in the measurement due to instrument calibration, ambient temperature etc.

Subjective and objective measurements

The characteristics of subjective and objective measurements are shown in Table 3.2. Measurements are described as being *subjective* when they are open to interpretation by the subject or the observer. Examples of subjective measurements include questionnaires that collect information such as symptom severity or frequency, quality of life, or satisfaction with medical services using coded responses or scores. When questionnaires are administered by the research staff rather than being self-administered by the subjects themselves, blinding and training are important practices that reduce observer bias. Poor between-observer agreement for subjective assessments can make it very difficult to make between-group comparisons when different observers are used, or to compare the results from studies conducted by different research groups.[1]

Table 3.2   Subjective and objective measurements
Subjective measurements • can be a subject report or a researcher observation • are prone to inconsistency and observer bias • collect information that may be similar to that collected in a clinical situation • time is not a problem so that retrospective information can be collected in addition to current information • ask questions of importance to the patient
Objective measurements • are measured by an observer (blinded or unblinded) • are often more precise than subjective measurements • can include archival data • ideal for measuring short-term conditions at a single point in time, such as X-rays, blood pressure, or lung function • preferable as the main study outcomes because the potential for bias is reduced

The inherent disadvantage with questionnaires is that they only provide subjective information, but this is balanced by the advantage that they are a cheap and efficient method of collecting information that is relevant to the subject, and for which the time of events is not a problem. For this reason, clinical trials in which the most important outcome is whether the patient feels better use self-reported health status as the primary outcome. In many research situations, such as in community studies, questionnaires are the only instruments that can be used to collect information of illness severity and history.

In contrast, *objective* measurements are collected by instruments that are less easily open to interpretation or to influence by the subject or the observer. Examples of objective measurements include those of physiology, biochemistry or radiology measured by laboratory or clinical equipment. Objective measurements have the advantage that they reduce observer and measurement bias. However, these types of measurements also have the disadvantage that, in general, they only collect short-term information such as lung function or blood pressure at the time of data collection, and they usually require contact with the subject, which may reduce the response rate for study.

Because objective measurements are less prone to observer and reporting bias than subjective measurements, they are preferred for testing the main study hypotheses. Some examples in which subjective questionnaire measurements can be replaced by objective outcome measurements are shown in Table 3.3.

Table 3.3 Examples of subjective and objective outcome measurements
Example 1 Subjective: 'Do you ever forget to take the capsules?' Objective: Counts of returned capsules or biochemical tests
Example 2 Subjective: 'How mobile is your child?' Objective: Tracking of movements with a mobility monitor
Example 3 Subjective: 'Has your chest felt tight or wheezy in the last week?' Objective: Lung function tests or peak flow meter readings

Responsiveness

In trials to measure the efficacy or effectiveness of an intervention, it is crucial that the main outcome measurement is responsive to essential differences between subjects or to changes that occur within a subject. In common with measuring validity and repeatability, methodology studies to demonstrate that an instrument is responsive to clinically important within-subject changes need to be designed and conducted appropriately.[2, 3] Methods for measuring responsiveness are based on comparing the minimum clinically important difference indicated by the measurement to the variability in stable subjects over time.[4, 5]

Many measurements are inherently unresponsive to small changes in disease severity and are not suitable for use as primary outcome variables in studies designed to document the effects of treatment or environmental interventions. For example, measurements such as a 5-point score in which symptom frequency is categorised as 'constant, frequent, occasional, rare or never' are not responsive for measuring subtle changes in symptom frequency or severity. When using scales such as this, it is quite unlikely that any new treatment or intervention would improve symptom frequency by an entire category in most subjects. To increase the responsiveness of this type of scale, the range would need to be lengthened by adding subcategories between the main scores.

In estimating which subjects are most likely to benefit from a treatment, it may be important to include measurements of quality of life and symptom or functional status. These outcomes may identify within-subject changes that are small but that are important to the patient.[6] In this way, the proportion of subjects who experience an improvement in their illness that has a positive impact on their quality of life can be estimated. Inclusion of these types of outcomes often provides more clinically relevant information than measures of physiological parameters that may not reflect the importance of the clinical condition to the patient.

Multiple outcome measurements

Many studies use multiple outcome measurements in order to collect comprehensive data. This is common when efficacy or effectiveness needs to be measured across a broad range of clinical outcomes. If this approach is used, then methods to avoid inaccurate reporting are essential. Such methods include specification of the primary and secondary outcome variables before the study begins, corrections for multiple testing, combining several outcomes into a single severity score, or using a combined outcome such as time to first event.[7]

It is essential that a study has the power to test the most important outcomes (Example 3.1). In practice, a single outcome measurement will rarely be adequate to assess the risks, costs and diverse benefits that may arise from the use of a new intervention.[8] For example, in the randomised trial shown in Example 2.1 in Chapter 2, the efficacy of the drug dexamethasone was evaluated in children with bacterial meningitis. In this study, the many outcome measurements included days of fever, presence of neurological abnormalities, severity scores, biochemical markers of cerebrospinal fluid, white cell counts, hearing impairment indicators and death.[9] Without the collection of all of these data, any important benefits or harmful effects of the drug regime may not have been documented.

Example 3.1   Use of alternate outcome measurements

A meta-analysis of the results of thirteen studies that investigated the use of aminophylline in the emergency treatment of asthma was reported in 1988.[10] This meta-analysis concluded that aminophylline was not effective in the treatment for severe, acute asthma in a hospital emergency situation because it did not result in greater improvements in spirometric measurements when compared to other bronchodilators. However, a later randomised controlled trial found that the use of aminophylline decreased the rate of hospital admissions of patients presenting to emergency departments with acute asthma.[11] In the former studies, the use of spirometric measurements may have been an inappropriate outcome measurement to estimate the efficacy of aminophylline in an emergency situation because spirometric function is of less importance to most patients and hospital managers than avoiding hospitalisation and returning home and to normal function.

When designing a study, it is important to remember that the outcomes that are significant to the subjects may be different from the outcomes that are significant to clinical practice. For example, a primary interest of clinicians may be to reduce hospital admissions whereas a primary interest of the subject may be to return to work or school, or to be able to exercise regularly. To avoid under-estimating the benefits of new interventions in terms of health aspects that are important to patients, both types of outcomes need to be included in the study design.[12] In studies in which children or dependent subjects are enrolled, indicators of the impact of disease on the family and carers must be measured in addition to measurements that are indicators of health status.

Impact on sample size requirements

Statistical power is always a major consideration when choosing outcome measurements. The problems of making decisions about a sample size that balances statistical power with clinical importance are discussed in more detail in Chapter 4.

In general, continuously distributed measurements provide greater statistical power for the same sample size than categorical measurements. For example, a measurement such as blood pressure on presentation has a continuous distribution. This measurement will provide greater statistical power for the same sample size than if the number of subjects with an abnormally high blood pressure is used as the outcome variable. Also, if a categorical variable is used, then a larger sample size will be required to show the same absolute difference between groups for a condition that occurs infrequently than for a condition that occurs frequently.

In any study, the sample size must be adequate to demonstrate that a clinically important difference between groups in all outcome measurements is statistically significant. Although it is common practice to calculate the sample size for a study using only the primary outcome measurements, this should not leave the findings unclear for other important secondary outcome measurements. This can arise if a secondary outcome variable occurs with a lower frequency in the study population or has a wider standard deviation than the primary outcome variable. Provided that the sample size is adequate, studies in which a wide range of outcome measurements is used are usually more informative and lead to a better comparability of the results with other studies than studies in which only a single categorical outcome measurement is used.

Surrogate end-points

In long-term clinical trials, the primary outcome variable is often called an *end-point*. This end-point may be a more serious but less frequent outcome, such as mortality, that is of primary importance to clinical practice. In contrast, variables that are measured and used as the primary outcome variable in interim analyses conducted before the study is finished are called *surrogate end-points*, or are sometimes called *alternative short-term outcomes*.

The features of surrogate outcome measurements are shown in Table 3.4. Surrogate outcomes may include factors that are important for determining mechanisms, such as blood pressure or cholesterol level as a surrogate for heart disease, or bone mineral density as a surrogate for bone fractures. For example, the extent of tumour shrinkage after some weeks of treatment may be used as a surrogate for survival rates over a period of years. In addition, surrogate outcomes may include lifestyle factors that are important to the patient, such as cost, symptom severity, side effects and quality of life. The use of these outcomes is essential for the evaluation of new drug therapies. However, it is important to be cautious about the results of interim analyses of surrogate outcomes because apparent benefits of therapies may be overturned in later analyses based on the primary end-points that have a major clinical impact.[13]

Table 3.4   Features of surrogate outcome measurements

- reduce sample size requirements and follow-up time
- may be measures of physiology or quality of life rather than measures of clinical importance
- useful for short-term, interim analyses
- only reliable if causally related to the outcome variable
- may produce unnecessarily pessimistic or optimistic results

Because the actual mechanisms of action of a clinical intervention cannot be anticipated, only the primary outcome should be regarded as the true clinical outcome. The practice of conducting interim analyses of surrogate outcomes is only valid in situations in which the surrogate variable can reliably predict the primary clinical outcome. However, this is rarely the case.[14] For example, in a trial of a new treatment for AIDS, CD4 blood count was used as an outcome variable in the initial analyses but turned out to be a poor predictor of survival in later stages of the study and therefore was a poor surrogate end-point.[15]

Because clinical end-points are used to measure efficacy, they often require the long-term follow-up of the study subjects. The advantage of including surrogate outcomes in a trial is that they can be measured much more quickly than the long-term clinical outcomes so that some results of the study become available much earlier. Also, the use of several surrogate and primary outcome measurements make it possible to collect information of both the mechanisms of the treatment, which is of importance to researchers, and information of therapeutic outcomes, which is of importance to the patient and to clinicians. However, a treatment may not always act through the mechanisms identified by the surrogate. Also, the construct validity of the surrogate outcome as a predictor of clinical outcome can only be assessed in large clinical trials that achieve completion in terms of measuring their primary clinical indicators.

Section 2—Confounders and effect-modifiers

The objectives of this section are to understand how to:
- explore which variables cause bias;
- identify and distinguish confounders, effect-modifiers and intervening variables;
- reduce bias caused by confounding and effect-modification;
- use confounders and effect-modifiers in statistical analyses; and
- categorise variables for use in multivariate analyses

Measuring associations

In health research, we often strive to measure the effect of a treatment or of an exposure on a clinical outcome or the presence of disease. In deciding whether the effect that we measure is real, we need to be certain that it cannot be explained by an alternative factor. In any type of study, except for large randomised controlled trials, it is possible for the measure of association between a disease or an outcome and an exposure or treatment to be altered by nuisance factors called confounders or effect-modifiers. These factors cause bias because their effects get mixed together with the effects of the factors being investigated.

Confounders and effect-modifiers are one of the major considerations in designing a research study. Because these factors can lead to a serious under-estimation or over-estimation of associations, their effects need to be taken into account either in the study design or in the data analyses.

Glossary

Term	Meaning
Bias	Distortion of the association between two factors
Under-estimation	Finding a weaker association between two variables than actually exists
Over-estimation	Finding a stronger association between two variables than actually exists

The essential characteristics of confounders and effect-modifiers are shown in Table 3.5. Because of their potential to influence the results, the effects of confounders and effect-modifiers must be carefully considered and minimised at both the study design and the data analysis stages of all research studies. These factors, both of which are related to the exposure being measured, are sometimes called *co-variates*.

Table 3.5   Characteristics of confounders and effect-modifiers

Confounders
- are a nuisance effect that needs to be removed
- are established risk factors for the outcome of interest
- cause a bias that needs to be minimised
- are not on the causal pathway between the exposure and outcome
- their effect is usually caused by selection or allocation bias
- should not be identified using a significance test
- must be controlled for in the study design or data analyses

Effect-modifiers
- change the magnitude of the relationship between two other variables
- interact in the causal pathway between an exposure and outcome
- have an effect that is independent of the study design and that is not caused by selection or allocation bias
- can be identified using a significance test
- need to be described in the data analyses

Confounders

Confounders are factors that are associated with both the outcome and the exposure but that are not directly on the causal pathway. Figure 3.1 shows how a confounder is an independent risk factor for the outcome of interest and is also independently related to the exposure of interest. Confounding is a potential problem in all studies except large, randomised controlled trials. Because of this, both the direction and the magnitude of the effects of confounders need to be investigated. In extreme cases, adjusting for the effects of a confounder may actually change the direction of the observed effect between an exposure and an outcome.

Figure 3.1   Relation of a confounder to the exposure and the outcome

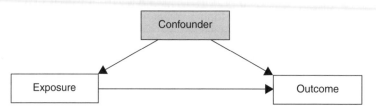

An example of a confounder is a history of smoking in the relationship between heart disease and exercise habits. A history of smoking is a risk factor for heart disease, irrespective of exercise frequency, but is also associated with exercise frequency in that the prevalence of smoking is generally lower in people who exercise regularly. This is a typical example of how, in epidemiological studies, the effects of confounders often result from subjects self-selecting themselves into related exposure groups.

The decision to regard a factor as a confounder should be based on clinical plausibility and prior evidence, and not on statistical significance. In practice, adjusting for an established confounder increases both the efficiency and the credibility of a study. However, the influence of a confounder only needs to be considered if its effect on the association being studied is large enough to be of clinical importance. In general, it is less important to adjust for the influence of confounders that have a small effect that becomes statistically significant as a result of a large sample size, because they have a minimal influence on results. However, it is always important to adjust for confounders that have a substantial influence, say with an odds ratio of 2.0 or greater, even if their effect is not statistically significant because the sample size is relatively small.

In randomised controlled trials, confounders are often measured as baseline characteristics. It is not usual to adjust for differences in baseline characteristics between groups that have arisen by chance. It is only necessary to make a mathematical adjustment for confounders in randomised controlled trials in which the difference in the distribution of a confounder between groups is large and in which the confounder is strongly related to the outcome.

An example of a study in which the effect of parental smoking as a confounder for many illness outcomes in childhood was measured is shown in Example 3.2. If studies of the aetiology or prevention of any of the outcome conditions in childhood are conducted in the future, the effects of parental smoking on the measured association will need to be considered. This could be achieved by randomly allocating children to study groups or by measuring the presence of parental smoking and adjusting for this effect in the data analyses.

Example 3.2 Study of confounding factors	
Burke et al. Parental smoking and risk factors for cardiovascular disease in 10–12 year old children[16]	
Characteristic	**Description**
Aims	To examine whether parent's health behaviours influence their children's health behaviours
Type of study	Cross-sectional
Sample base	Year 6 students from 18 randomly chosen schools
Subjects	804 children (81%) who consented to participate
Outcome measurements	Dietary intake by mid-week 2-day diet record; out-of-school physical activity time by 7-day diaries; smoking behaviour by questionnaire; height, weight, waist and hip circumference, skin fold thickness
Statistics	Multiple regression
Conclusion	• parental smoking is a risk factor for lower physical activity, more television watching, fat intake, body mass index and waist-to-hip ratio in children • studies to examine these outcomes will need to take exposure to parental smoking into account
Strengths	• large population sample enrolled therefore good generalisability within selection criteria and effects quantified with precision • objective anthropometric measurements used
Limitations	• size of risk factors not quantified as adjusted odds ratios • R^2 value from regression analyses not included so that the amount of variation explained is not known • results cannot be generalised outside the restricted age range of subjects • no information of other known confounders such as height or weight of parents collected • possibility of effect modification not explored

Effect of selection bias on confounding

Confounders become a major problem when they are distributed unevenly in the treatment and control groups, or in the exposed and unexposed groups. This usually occurs as a result of selection bias, for example in clinical studies when subjects self-select themselves into a control or treatment group rather than being randomly assigned to a group. Selection bias also occurs in epidemiological studies when subjects self-select themselves into a related exposure group. In the example shown in Figure 3.2, smokers have self-selected themselves into a low exercise frequency group. When this happens, the presence of the confounding factor (smoking status) will lead to an under-estimation or over-estimation of the association between the outcome (heart disease) and the exposure under investigation (low exercise frequency).

Figure 3.2   Role of smoking as a confounder in the relation between regular exercise and heart disease

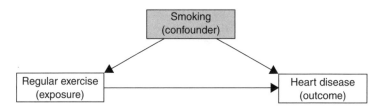

Using random allocation to control for confounding

The major advantage of randomised controlled trials is that confounders that are both known and unknown will be, by chance, distributed evenly between the intervention and control groups if the sample size is large enough. In fact, randomisation is the only method by which both the measured and unmeasured confounders can be controlled. Because the distribution of confounders is balanced between groups in these studies, their effects do not need to be taken into account in the analyses.

Glossary

Term	Meaning
Randomisation	Allocating subjects randomly to the treatment, intervention or control groups
Restriction	Restricting the sampling criteria or data analyses to a subset of the sample, such as all females
Matching	Choosing controls that match the cases on important confounders such as age or gender
Multivariate analyses	Statistical method to adjust the exposure–outcome relationships for the effects of one or more confounders
Stratification	Dividing the sample into small groups according to a confounder such as ethnicity or gender

Testing for confounding

When there are only two categories of exposure for the confounder, the outcome and the exposure variable, the presence of confounding can be tested using stratified analyses. If the stratified estimates are different from the estimate in the total sample, this indicates that the effects of confounding are present. An example of the results from a study designed to measure the relationship between chronic bronchitis and area of residence in which smoking was a confounder are shown in Table 3.6.

Table 3.6 Testing for the effects of confounding		
Sample	Comparison	Relative risk for having chronic bronchitis
Total sample	Urban vs rural	1.5 (95% CI 1.1, 1.9)
Non-smokers	Urban vs rural	1.2 (95% CI 0.6, 2.2)
Smokers	Urban vs rural	1.2 (95% CI 0.9, 1.6)

In the total sample, living in an urban area was a significant risk factor for having chronic bronchitis because the 95 per cent confidence interval around the relative risk of 1.5 does not encompass the value of unity. However, the effect is reduced when examined in the non-smokers and smokers separately. The lack of significance in the two strata examined separately is a function of the relative risk being reduced from 1.5 to 1.2, and the fact that the sample size is smaller in each strata than in the total sample. Thus, the reduction from a relative risk of 1.5 to 1.2 is attributable to the presence of smoking, which is a confounder in the relation between rural residence and chronic bronchitis.[17] We can surmise that the prevalence of smoking, which explains the apparent urban–rural difference, is much higher in the urban region.

If the effect of confounding had not been taken into account, the relationship between chronic bronchitis and region of residence would have been over-estimated. The relation between the three variables being studied in this example is shown in Figure 3.3.

Figure 3.3   Relation of a confounder (smoking history) to the exposure (urban residence) and the outcome (chronic bronchitis)

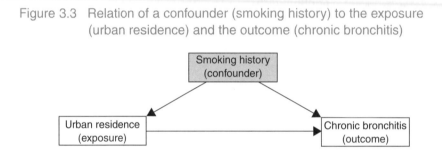

Adjusting for the effects of confounders

Removing the effects of confounding can be achieved at the design stage of the study, which is preferable, or at the data analysis stage, which is less satisfactory. The use of randomisation at the recruitment stage of a study will ensure that the distribution of confounders is balanced between each of the study groups, as long as the sample size is large enough. If potential confounders are evenly distributed in the treatment and non-treatment groups then the bias is minimised and no further adjustment is necessary. The methods that can be used to control for the effects of confounders are shown in Table 3.7.

Clearly, it is preferable to control for the effects of confounding at the study design stage. This is particularly important in case-control and cohort studies in which selection bias can cause an uneven distribution of confounders between the study groups. Cross-sectional studies and ecological studies are also particularly vulnerable to the effects of confounding. Several methods, including restriction, matching and stratification, can be used to control for known confounders in these types of studies.

Table 3.7	Methods of reducing the effects of confounders in order of merit

Study design
- randomise to control for known and unknown confounders
- restrict subject eligibility using inclusion and exclusion criteria
- select subjects by matching for major confounders
- stratify subject selection, e.g. select males and females separately

Data analysis
- demonstrate comparability of confounders between study groups
- stratify analyses by the confounder
- use multivariate analyses to adjust for confounding

Compensation for confounding at the data analysis stage is less effective than randomising in the design stage, because the adjustment may be incomplete, and is also less efficient because a larger sample size is required. To adjust for the effects of confounders at the data analysis stage requires that the sample size is large enough and that adequate data have been collected. One approach is to conduct analyses by different levels or strata of the confounder, for example by conducting separate analyses for each gender or for different age groups. The problem with this approach is that the statistical power is significantly reduced each time the sample is stratified or divided.

The effects of confounders are often minimised by adjustments in multivariate or logistic regression analyses. Because these methods use a mathematical adjustment rather than efficient control in the study design, they are the least effective method of controlling for confounding. However, multivariate analyses have the practical advantage over stratification in that they retain statistical power, and therefore increase precision, and they allow for the control of several confounders at one time.

Effect-modifiers

Effect-modifiers, as the name indicates, are factors that modify the effect of a causal factor on an outcome of interest. Effect-modifiers are sometimes described as *interacting variables*. The way in which an effect-modifier operates is shown in Figure 3.4. Effect-modifiers can often be recognised because they have a different effect on the exposure–outcome relation in each of the strata being examined. A classic example of this is age, which modifies the effect of many disease conditions in that the risk of disease becomes increasingly greater with increasing age. Thus, if risk estimates are calculated for different age strata, the estimates become larger with each increasing increment of age category.

Figure 3.4   Relation of an effect-modifier to the exposure and the outcome

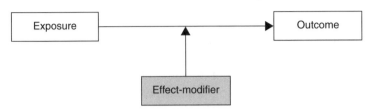

Effect-modifiers have a dose–response relationship with the outcome variable and, for this reason, are factors that can be described in stratified analyses, or by statistical interactions in multivariate analyses. If effect-modification is present, the sample size must be large enough to be able to describe the effect with precision.

Table 3.8 shows an example in which effect-modification is present. In this example, the risk of myocardial infarction is stronger, that is has a higher relative risk, in those who have normal blood pressure compared to those with high blood pressure when the sample is stratified by smoking status.[18] Thus blood pressure is acting as an effect-modifier in the relationship between smoking status and the risk of myocardial infarction. In this example, the risk of myocardial infarction is increased to a greater extent by smoking in subjects with normal blood pressure than in those with elevated blood pressure.

Table 3.8   Example in which the number of cigarettes smoked daily is an effect-modifier in the relation between blood pressure and the risk of myocardial infarction in a population sample of nurses[19]

| | Relative risk of myocardial infarction | |
Smoking status	Normal blood pressure	High blood pressure
Never smoked	1.0	1.0
1–14 per day	2.8 (1.5, 5.1)	1.4 (0.9, 2.2)
15–24 per day	5.0 (3.4, 7.3)	3.5 (2.4, 5.0)
25 or more per day	8.6 (5.8, 12.7)	2.8 (2.0, 3.9)

If effect-modification is present, then stratum specific measures of effect should be reported. However, it is usually impractical to describe more than a few effect-modifiers in this way. If two or more effect-modifiers are present, it is usually better to describe their effects using interaction terms in multivariate analyses.

Using multivariate analyses to describe confounders and effect-modifiers

Confounders and effect-modifiers are treated very differently from one another in multivariate analyses. For example, a multiple regression model can be used to adjust for the effects of confounders on outcomes that are continuously distributed. A model to predict lung function may take the form:

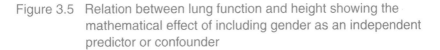

Lung function = Intercept + β1 (height) + β2 (gender)

where height is a confirmed explanatory variable and gender is the predictive variable of interest whose effect is being measured. An example of this type of relationship is shown in Figure 3.5 in which it can be seen that lung function depends on both height and gender but that gender is an independent risk factor, or a confounder, because the regression lines are parallel.

Figure 3.5 Relation between lung function and height showing the mathematical effect of including gender as an independent predictor or confounder

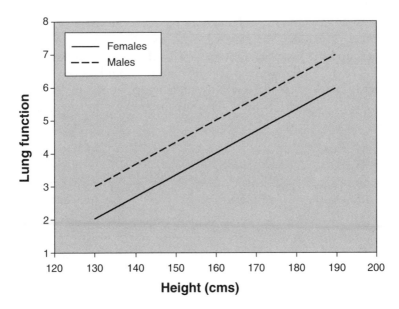

Health science research

Alternatively, a logistic regression model can be used to adjust for confounding when the outcome variable is categorical. A model for the data in the example shown in Table 3.2 would take the form:

$$\text{Risk of chronic bronchitis} = \begin{array}{c}\text{odds for}\\\text{urban residence}\end{array} \times \begin{array}{c}\text{odds for}\\\text{ever smoked}\end{array}$$

When developing these types of multivariate models, it is important to consider the size of the estimates, that is the β coefficients. The confounder (i.e. the gender or smoking history terms in the examples above) should always be included if its effects are significant in the model. The term should also be included if it is a documented risk factor and its effect in the model is not significant.

A potential confounder must also be included in the model when it is not statistically significant but its inclusion changes the size of the effect of other variables (such as height or residence in an urban region) by more than 5–10 per cent. An advantage of this approach is that its inclusion may reduce the standard error and thereby increase the precision of the estimate of the exposure of interest.[20] If the inclusion of a variable inflates the standard error substantially, then it probably shares a degree of collinearity with one of the other variables and should be omitted.

A more complex multiple regression model, which is needed to investigate whether gender is an effect-modifier that influences lung function, may take the form:

Lung function = Intercept + β1 (height) + β2 (gender) + β3 (height*gender)

An example of this type of relationship is described in Example 3.3. Figure 3.6 shows an example in which gender modifies the effect of height on lung function. In this case, the slopes are not parallel indicating that gender is an effect-modifier because it interacts with the relation between height and lung function. Similarly, the effect of smoking could be tested as an effect-modifier in the logistic regression example above by testing for the statistical significance of a multiplicative term urban*smoking in the model, i.e.:

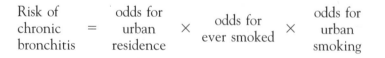

Suppose that, in this model, urban region is coded as 0 for non-urban and 1 for urban residence, and smoking history is coded as 0 for non-smokers and 1 for ever smoked. Then, the interaction term will be zero for all

Figure 3.6   Relation between lung function and height showing the
mathematical effect when gender is an effect-modifier
that interacts with height

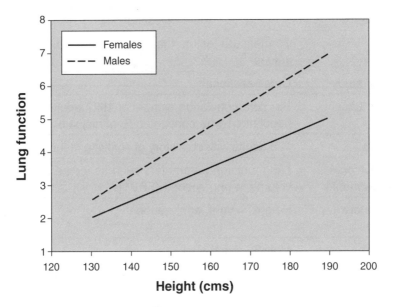

The two lines show the relation between lung function and height in males and females. The
slopes of the two lines show the mathematical effect of gender, an effect-modifier that
interacts with height to explain the explanatory and outcome variables.

subjects who are non-smokers and for all subjects who do not live in an
urban region, and will have the value of 1 for only the subjects who both
live in an urban region and who have ever smoked. In this way, the
additional risk in this group is estimated by multiplying the odds ratio for
the interaction term.

When testing for the effects of interactions, especially in studies in
which the outcome variable is dichotomous, up to four times as many subjects may be needed in order to gain the statistical power to test the interaction and describe its effects with precision. This can become a dilemma
when designing a clinical trial because a large sample size is really the only
way to test whether one treatment enhances or inhibits the effect of
another treatment, that is whether the two treatment effects interact with
one another. However, a larger sample size is not needed if no interactive
effect is present.

Example 3.3	Effect-modification
Belousova et al. Factors that effect normal lung function in white Australian adults[21]	
Characteristic	Description
Aims	To measure factors that predict normal lung function values
Type of study	Cross-sectional
Sample base	Random population sample of 1527 adults (61% of population) who consented to participate
Subjects	729 adults with no history of smoking or lung disease
Main outcome measurements	Lung function parameters such as forced expiratory volume in one second (FEV1)
Explanatory variables	Height, weight, age, gender
Statistics	Multiple regression
Conclusion	• normal values for FEV1 in Australian adults quantified • interaction found between age and male gender in that males had a greater decline in FEV1 with age than females after adjusting for height and weight • gender is an effect-modifier when describing FEV1
Strengths	• large population sample enrolled, therefore results generalisable to age range and effects quantified with precision • new reference values obtained
Limitations	• estimates may have been influenced by selection bias as a result of moderate response rate • misclassification bias, as a result groups being defined according to questionnaire data of smoking and symptom history, may have led to an underestimation of normal values

Intervening variables

Intervening variables are an alternate outcome of the exposure being investigated. The relationship between an exposure, an outcome and an intervening variable is shown in Figure 3.7.

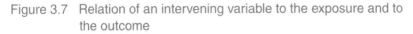
Figure 3.7 Relation of an intervening variable to the exposure and to the outcome

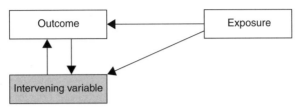

In any multivariate analysis, intervening variables, which are an alternative outcome of the exposure variable being investigated, cannot be included as exposure variables. Intervening variables have a large degree of collinearity with the outcome of interest and therefore they distort multivariate models because they share the same variation with the outcome variable that we are trying to explain with the exposure variables.

For example, in a study to measure the factors that influence the development of asthma, other allergic symptoms such as hay fever would be intervening variables because they are part of the same allergic process that leads to the development of asthma. This type of relationship between variables is shown in Figure 3.8. Because hay fever is an outcome of an allergic predisposition, hay fever and asthma have a strong association, or collinearity, with one another.

Figure 3.8 Example in which hay fever is an intervening variable in the relation between exposure to airborne particles, such as moulds or pollens, and symptoms of asthma

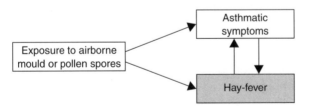

Distinguishing between confounders, effect-modifiers and intervening variables

The decision about whether risk factors are confounders, effect-modifiers or intervening variables requires careful consideration to measure their independent effects in the data analyses. The classification of variables also depends on a thorough knowledge of previous evidence about the determinants of the outcome being studied and the biological mechanisms that explain the relationships. The misinterpretation of the role of any of these variables will lead to bias in the study results. For example, if effect-modifiers are treated as confounders and controlled for in the study design, then the effect of the exposure of interest is likely to be underestimated and, because the additional interactive term is not included, important etiological information will be lost. Similarly, if an intervening variable is treated as an independent risk factor for a disease outcome, the information about other risk factors will be distorted.

Confounders, effect-modifiers and intervening variables can all be either categorical variables or continuously distributed measurements. Before undertaking any statistical analysis, the information that has been collected must be divided into outcome, intervening and explanatory variables as shown in Table 3.9. This will prevent errors that may distort the effects of the analyses and reduce the precision of the estimates.

Table 3.9	Categorisation of variables for data analysis and presentation of results	
Variable	**Subsets**	**Alternative names**
Outcome variables		Dependent variables (DVs)
Intervening variables		Secondary or alternative outcome variables
Explanatory variables	Confounders Effect-modifiers	Independent variables (IVs) Risk factors Predictors Exposure variables Prognostic factors Interactive variables

The effects of confounders and effect-modifiers are usually established from previously published studies and must be taken into account whether or not they are statistically significant in the sample. However, it is often difficult to determine whether effect-modification is present, especially if the sample size is quite small. For these reasons, careful study design and careful analysis of the data by researchers who have insight into the mechanisms of the development of the outcome are essential components of good research.

Section 3—Validity

The objectives of this section are to understand how to:
- improve the accuracy of a measurement instrument;
- design studies to measure validity; and
- decide whether the results from a study are reliable and generalisable.

Validity

Validity is an estimate of the accuracy of an instrument or of the study results. There are two distinct types of validity, that is internal validity which is the extent to which the study methods are reliable, and external validity which is the extent to which the study results can be applied to a wider population.

External validity

If the results of a clinical or population study can be applied to a wider population, then a study has external validity, that is good *generalisability*. The external validity of a study is a concept that is described rather than an association that is measured using statistical methods.

In clinical trials, the external validity must be strictly defined and can be maintained by adhering to the inclusion and exclusion criteria when enrolling the subjects. Violation of these criteria can make it difficult to identify the population group to whom the results apply.

Health science research

Clinical studies have good external validity if the subjects are recruited from hospital-based patients but the results can be applied to the general population in the region of the hospital. In population research, a study has good external validity if the subjects are selected using random sampling methods and if a high response rate is obtained so that the results are applicable to the entire population from which the study sample was recruited, and to other similar populations.

Internal validity

A study has internal validity if its measurements and methods are accurate and repeatable, that is if the measurements are a good estimate of what they are expected to measure and if the within-subject and between-observer errors are small. If a study has good internal validity, any differences in measurements between the study groups can be attributed solely to the hypothesised effect under investigation. The types of internal validity that can be measured are shown in Table 3.10.

Table 3.10 Internal validity		
Type	Subsets	Meaning
Face validity	Measurement validity Internal consistency	Extent to which a method measures what it is intended to measure
Content validity		Extent to which questionnaire items cover the research area of interest
Criterion validity	Predictive utility Concurrent validity Diagnostic utility	Agreement with a 'gold standard'
Construct validity	Criterion-related validity Convergent validity Discriminant validity	Agreement with other tests

An important concept of validity is that it is an estimate of the accuracy of a test in measuring what we want it to measure. Internal validity of an instrument is largely situation specific; that is, it only applies to similar subjects studied in a similar setting.[22] In general, the concept of internal validity is not as essential for objective physical measurements, such as scales to measure weight or spirometers to measure lung function. However, information of internal validity is essential in situations where a measurement is being used as a practical surrogate for another more precise instrument, or is being used to predict a disease or an outcome at some time in the future. For example, it may be important to know the validity of measurements of blood pressure as indicators of the presence of current cardiovascular disease, or predictors of the future development of cardiovascular disease.

Information about internal validity is particularly important when subjective measurements, that is measurements that depend on personal responses to questions, such as those of previous symptom history, quality of life, perception of pain or psychosocial factors, are being used. Responses to these questions may be biased by many factors including lifetime experience and recognition or understanding of the terms being used. Obviously, instruments that improve internal validity by reducing measurement bias are more valuable as both research and clinical tools.

If a new questionnaire or instrument is being devised then its internal validity has to be established so that confidence can be placed on the information that is collected. Internal validity also needs to be established if an instrument is used in a research setting or in a group of subjects in which it has not previously been validated. The development of scientific and research instruments often requires extensive and ongoing collection of data and can be quite time consuming, but the process often leads to new and valuable types of information.

Glossary

Term	Meaning
Items	Individual questions in a questionnaire
Constructs	Underlying factors that cannot be measured directly, e.g. anxiety or depression, which are measured indirectly by the expression of several symptoms or behaviours
Domain	A group of several questions that together estimate a single subject characteristic, or construct
Instrument	Questionnaire or piece of equipment used to collect outcome or exposure measurements
Generalisability	Extent to which the study results can be applied in a wider community setting

Face validity

Face validity, which is sometimes called *measurement validity*, is the extent to which a method measures what it is intended to measure. For subjective instruments such as questionnaires, validity is usually assessed by the judgment of an expert panel rather than by the use of formal statistical methods. Good face validity is essential because it is a measure of the expert perception of the acceptance, appropriateness and precision of an instrument or questionnaire. This type of validity is therefore an estimate of the extent to which an instrument or questionnaire fulfils its purpose in collecting accurate information about the characteristics, diseases or exposures of a subject. As such, face validity is an assessment of the degree of confidence that can be placed on inferences from studies that have used the instrument in question.

When designing a questionnaire, relevant questions increase face validity because they increase acceptability whereas questions that are not answered because they appear irrelevant decrease face validity. The face validity of a questionnaire also decreases if replies to some questions are easily falsified by subjects who want to appear better or worse than they actually are.

Face validity can be improved by making clear decisions about the nature and the purpose of the instrument, and by an expert panel reaching a consensus opinion about both the content and wording of the questions. It is important that questions make sense intuitively to both the researchers and to the subjects, and that they provide a reasonable approach in the face of current knowledge.

Content validity

Content validity is the extent to which the items in a questionnaire adequately cover the domain under investigation. This term is also used to describe the extent to which a measurement quantifies what we want it to measure. As with face validity, this is also a concept that is judged by experts rather than by being judged by using formal statistical analyses. The methods to increase content validity are shown in Table 3.11.

Within any questionnaire, each question will usually have a different content validity. For example, questionnaire responses by parents about whether their child was hospitalised for a respiratory infection in early life will have better content validity than responses to questions about the occurrence of respiratory infections in later childhood that did not require hospitalisation. Hospitalisation in early childhood is a more traumatic event that has a greater impact on the family. Thus, this question will be subject to less recall or misclassification bias than that of less serious infections

Table 3.11   Methods to increase content validity
• the presence and the severity of the disease are both assessed • all characteristics relevant to the disease of interest are covered • the questionnaire is comprehensive in that no important areas are missed • the questions measure the entire range of circumstances of an exposure • all known confounders are measured

that can be treated by a general practitioner and may have been labelled as one of many different respiratory conditions.

When developing a questionnaire that has many items, it can be difficult to decide which items to maintain or to eliminate. In doing this, it is often useful to perform a factor analysis to determine which questions give replies that cluster together to measure symptoms of the same illness or exposure, and which belong to an independent domain. This type of analysis provides a better understanding of the instrument and of replies to items that can either be omitted from the questionnaire, or that can be grouped together in the analyses. If a score is being developed, this process is also helpful for defining the weights that should be given to the items that contribute to the score.

In addition, an analysis of internal consistency (such as the statistical test Cronbach's alpha) can help to determine the extent to which replies to different questions address the same dimension because they elicit closely related replies. Eliminating items that do not correlate with each other increases internal consistency. However, this approach will lead to a questionnaire that only covers a limited range of domains and therefore has a restricted value. In general, it is usually better to sacrifice internal consistency for content validity, that is to maintain a broad scope by including questions that are both comprehensive in the information they obtain and are easily understood.

The content validity of objective measuring instruments also needs to be considered. For example, a single peak flow measurement has good content validity for measuring airflow limitation at a specific point in time when it can be compared to baseline levels that have been regularly monitored at some point in the past.[23] However, a single peak flow measurement taken alone has poor content validity for assessing asthma severity. In isolation, this measurement does not give any indication of the extent of day-to-day peak flow variability, airway narrowing or airway inflammation, or other factors that also contribute to the severity of the disease.

Criterion validity

Criterion validity is the extent to which a test agrees with a gold standard. It is essential that criterion validity is assessed when a less expensive, less time consuming, less invasive or more convenient test is being developed. If the new instrument or questionnaire provides a more accurate estimate of disease or of risk, or is more repeatable, more practical or more cost effective to administer than the current 'best' method, then it may replace this method. If the measurements from each instrument have a high level of agreement, they can be used interchangeably.

The study design for measuring criterion validity is shown in Table 3.12. In such studies, it is essential that the subjects are selected to give the entire range of measurements that can be encountered and that the test under consideration and the gold standard are measured independently and in consistent circumstances. The statistical methods that are used to describe criterion validity, which are called *methods of agreement*, are described in Chapter 7.

Table 3.12   Study design for measuring criterion and construct validity

- the conditions in which the two assessments are made are identical
- the order of the tests is randomised
- both the subject and the observer are blinded to the results of the first test
- a new treatment or clinical intervention is not introduced in the period between the two assessments
- the time between assessments is short enough so that the severity of the condition being measured has not changed

---

Predictive utility is a term that is sometimes used to describe the ability of a questionnaire to predict the gold standard test result at some time in the future. Predictive utility is assessed by administering a questionnaire and then waiting for an expected outcome to develop. For example, it may be important to measure the utility of questions of the severity of back pain in predicting future chronic back problems. In this situation, questions of pain history may be administered to a cohort of patients attending physiotherapy and then validated against whether the pain resolves or is ongoing at a later point in time. The predictive utility of a diagnostic tool can also be validated against later objective tests, for example against biochemical tests or X-ray results.

Construct validity

Construct validity is the extent to which a test agrees with another test in a way that is expected, or the extent to which a questionnaire predicts a disease that is classified using an objective measurement or diagnostic test, and is measured in situations when a gold standard is not available. In different disciplines, construct validity may be called *diagnostic utility*, *criterion-related* or *convergent validity*, or *concurrent validity*.

Example 3.4   Construct validity
Haftel et al. Hanging leg weight—a rapid technique for estimating total body weight in pediatric resuscitation[24]

Characteristic	Description
Aims	To validate measurements of estimating total body weight in children who cannot be weighed by usual weight scales
Type of study	Methodological
Subjects	100 children undergoing anesthesia
Outcome measurements	Total body weight, supine body length and hanging leg weight
Statistics	Regression models and correlation statistics
Conclusion	• Hanging leg weight is a better predictor of total body weight than is supine body length • Hanging leg weight takes less than 30 seconds and involves minimal intervention to head, neck or trunk regions
Strengths	• wide distribution of body weight distribution (4.4–47.5 kg) and age range (2–180 months) in the sample ensures generalisability • 'gold standard' available so criterion validity can be assessed
Limitations	• unclear whether observers measuring hanging leg weight were blinded to total body weight and supine body length • conclusions about lack of accuracy in children less than 10 kg not valid—less than 6 children fell into this group so validity not established for this age range

New instruments (or constructs) usually need to be developed when an appropriate instrument is not available or when the available instrument does not measure some key aspects. Thus, construct validity is usually measured during the development of a new instrument that is thought to be better in terms of the range it can measure or in its accuracy in predicting a disease, an exposure or a behaviour. The conditions under which construct validity is measured are the same as for criterion validity and are summarised in Table 3.12. An example of a study in which construct validity was assessed is shown in Example 3.4.

Construct validity is important for learning more about diseases and for increasing knowledge about both the theory of causation and the measure at the same time. Poor construct validity may result from difficult wording in a questionnaire, a restricted scale of measurement or a faulty construct. If construct validity is poor, the new instrument may be good but the theory about its relationship with the 'best available' method may be incorrect. Alternatively, the theory may be sound but the instrument may be a poor tool for discriminating the disease condition in question.

To reduce bias in any research study, both criterion and construct validity of the research instruments must already have been established in a sample of subjects who are representative of the study subjects in whom the instrument will be used.

Measuring validity

Construct and criterion validity are sometimes measured by recruiting extreme groups, that is subjects with a clinically recognised disorder and subjects who are well defined, healthy subjects. This may be a reasonable approach if the instrument will only be used in a specialised clinical setting. However, in practice, it is often useful to have an instrument that can discriminate disease not only in clearly defined subjects but also in the group in between who may not have the disorder or who have symptoms that are less severe and therefore characterise the disease with less certainty. The practice of selecting well-defined groups also suggests that an instrument that can discriminate between the groups is already available. If this approach is used, then the estimates of sensitivity and specificity will be over-estimated, and therefore will suggest better predictive power than if validity was measured in a random population sample.

The statistical methods used for assessing different types of validity are shown in Table 3.13 and are discussed in more detail in Chapter 7. No single study can be used to measure all types of validity, and the design of the study must be appropriate for testing the type of validity in question. When a gold standard is not available or is impractical to measure, the development of a better instrument is usually an ongoing process that involves several stages and a series of studies to establish both validity and repeatability. This process ensures that a measurement is both stable and precise, and therefore that it is reliable for accurately measuring what we want it to measure.

Table 3.13 Methods for assessing validity			
Type of validity	Sub-categories	Type of measurement	Analyses
External validity		Categorical or continuous	Sensitivity analyses Subjective judgments
Internal validity	Face and content validity	Categorical or continuous	Judged by experts Factor analysis Cronbach's alpha
	Criterion and construct validity	Both categorical	Sensitivity Specificity Predictive power Likelihood ratio Logistic regression
		Continuous to predict categorical	ROC curves
		Both continuous and the units the same	Measurement error ICC Mean-vs-differences plot
		Both continuous and the units different	Linear or multiple regression

Relation between validity and repeatability

Validity should not be confused with repeatability, which is an assessment of the precision of an instrument. In any research study, both the validity and the repeatability of the instruments used should have been established before data collection begins.

Measurements of repeatability are based on administering the instrument to the same subjects on two different occasions and then calculating the range in which the patient's 'true' measurement is likely to lie. An important concept is that a measurement with poor repeatability cannot have good validity but that criterion or construct validity is maximised if repeatability is high. On the other hand, good repeatability does not guarantee good validity although the maximum possible validity will be higher in instruments that have a good repeatability.

Section 4—Questionnaires and data forms

The objectives of this section are to understand:
- why questionnaires are used;
- how to design a questionnaire or a data collection form;
- why some questions are better than others;
- how to develop measurement scales; and
- how to improve repeatability and validity.

Developing a questionnaire

Most research studies use questionnaires to collect information about demographic characteristics and about previous and current illness symptoms, treatments and exposures of the subjects. A questionnaire has the advantage over objective measurement tools in that it is simple and cheap to administer and can be used to collect information about past as well as present symptoms. However, a reliable and valid questionnaire takes a long time and extensive resources to test and develop. It is important to remember that a questionnaire that is well designed not only has good face, content, and construct or criterion validity but also contributes to more efficient research and to greater generalisability of the results by minimising missing, invalid and unusable data.

The most important aspects to consider when developing a questionnaire are the presentation, the mode of administration and the content. The questionnaires that are most useful in research studies are those that have good content validity, and that have questions that are highly repeatable and responsive to detecting changes in subjects over time. Because repeatability, validity and responsiveness are determined by factors such as the types of questions and their wording and the sequence and the overall format, it is essential to pay attention to all of these aspects before using a questionnaire in a research study.

New questionnaires must be tested in a rigorous way before a study begins. The questionnaire may be changed several times during the pilot stage but, for consistency in the data, the questionnaire cannot be altered once the study is underway. The checklist steps for developing a questionnaire are shown in Table 3.14.

Table 3.14   Checklist for developing a new questionnaire
❑ Decide on outcome, explanatory and demographic data to be collected
❑ Search the literature for existing questionnaires
❑ Compile new and existing questions in a logical order
❑ Put the most important questions at the top
❑ Group questions into topics and order in a logical flow
❑ Decide whether to use categories or scales for replies
❑ Reach a consensus with co-workers and experts
❑ Simplify the wording and shorten as far as possible
❑ Decide on a coding schedule
❑ Conduct a pilot study
❑ Refine the questions and the formatting as often as necessary
❑ Test repeatability and establish validity

Mode of administration

Before deciding on the content of a questionnaire, it is important to decide on the mode of administration that will be used. Questionnaires may be self-administered, that is completed by the subject, or researcher-administered, that is the questions are asked and the questionnaire filled in by the researcher. In any research study, the data collection procedures must be standardised so that the conditions or the mode of administration remain constant throughout. This will reduce bias and increase internal validity.

In general, *self-administered* questionnaires have the advantage of being more easily standardised and of being economical in that they can be administered with efficiency in studies with a larger sample size. However, the response rate to self-administered questionnaires may be low and the use of these types of questionnaires does not allow for opportunities to clarify responses. In large population studies, such as registers of rare diseases, the physicians who are responsible for identifying the cases often complete the questionnaires.

On the other hand, *interviewer-administered* questionnaires, which can be face-to-face or over the telephone, have the advantages of being able to collect more complex information and of being able to minimise missing data. This type of data collection is more expensive and interviewer bias in interpreting responses can be a problem, but the method allows for greater flexibility.

Choosing the questions

The first step in designing a questionnaire is to conduct searches of the literature to investigate whether an appropriate, validated questionnaire or any other questionnaires with useful items is already available. Established questionnaires may exist but may not be helpful if the language is inappropriate for the setting or if critical questions are not included.

The most reliable questionnaires are those that are easily understood, that have a meaning that is the same to the researcher and to the respondent, and that are relevant to the research topic. When administering questionnaires in the community, even simple questions about gender, marital status and country of birth can collect erroneous replies.[25] Because replies can be inconsistent, it is essential that more complex questions about health outcomes and environmental exposures that are needed for testing the study hypotheses are as simple and as unambiguous as possible.

The differences between open-ended and closed-ended questions are shown in Table 3.15. Open-ended questions, which are difficult to code and analyse, should only be included when the purpose of the study is to develop new hypotheses or collect information on new topics.

If young children are being surveyed, parents need to complete the questionnaire but this means that information can only be obtained about visible signs and symptoms and not about feelings or less certain illnesses such as headaches, sensations of chest tightness etc.

A questionnaire that measures all of the information required in the study, including the outcomes, exposures, confounders and the demographic information, is an efficient research tool. To achieve this, questions that are often used in clinical situations or that are widely used in established questionnaires, such as the census forms, can be included. Another method for collating appropriate questions is to conduct a focus group to collect ideas about aspects of an illness or intervention that are important to the patient. Finally, peer review from people with a range of clinical and research experience is invaluable for refining the questionnaire.

Table 3.15   Differences between closed- and open-ended questions

Closed-ended questions and scales
- collect quantitative information
- provide fixed, often pre-coded, replies
- collect data quickly
- are easy to manage and to analyse
- validity is determined by choice of replies
- minimise observer bias
- may attract random responses

Open-ended questions
- collect qualitative information
- cannot be summarised in a quantitative way
- are often difficult and time consuming to summarise
- widen the scope of the information being collected
- elicit unprompted ideas
- are most useful when little is known about a research area
- are invaluable for developing new hypotheses

Sensitive questions

If sensitive information of ethnicity, income, family structure etc. is required, it is often a good idea to use the same wording and structure as the questions that are used in the national census. This saves the work of developing and testing the questions, and also provides a good basis for comparing the demographic characteristics of the study sample with those of the general population.

If the inclusion of sensitive questions will reduce the response rate, it may be a good idea to exclude the questions, especially if they are not essential for testing the hypotheses. Another alternative is to include them in an optional section at the end of the questionnaire.

Wording and layout

The characteristics of good research questions are shown in Table 3.16. The most useful questions usually have very simple sentence constructions that are easily understood. Questions should also be framed so that respondents can be expected to know the correct answer. A collection of questions with these characteristics is an invaluable research tool. An example of the layout of a questionnaire to collect various forms of quantitative information is shown in Table 3.22 at the end of this chapter.

Table 3.16   Characteristics of good research questions
• are relevant to the research topic
• are simple to answer and to analyse
• only ask one question per item
• cover all aspects of the illness or exposure being studied
• mean the same to the subject and to the researcher
• have good face, content and criterion or construct validity
• are highly repeatable
• are responsive to change

In general, positive wording is preferred because it prompts a more obvious response. 'Don't know' options should only be used if it is really possible that some subjects will not know the answer. In many situations, the inclusion of this option may invite evasion of the question and thereby increase the number of unusable responses. This results in inefficiency in the research project because a larger sample size will be required to answer the study question, and generalisability may be reduced.

When devising multi-response categories for replies, remember that they can be collapsed into combined groups later, but cannot be expanded should more detail be required. It is also important to decide how any missing data will be handled at the design stage of a study, for example whether missing data will be coded as negative responses or as missing variables. If missing data are coded as a negative response, then an instruction at the top of the questionnaire that indicates that the respondent should answer 'No' if the reply is uncertain can help to reduce the number of missing, and therefore ambiguous, replies.

To simplify the questions, ensure that they are not badly worded, ambiguous or irrelevant and do not use 'jargon' terms that are not universally understood. If subjects in a pilot study have problems understanding the questions, ask them to rephrase the question in their own words so that a more direct question can be formulated. Table 3.17 shows some examples of ambiguous questions and some alternatives that could be used.

Table 3.17 Ambiguous questions and alternatives that could be used

Ambiguous questions	Problem	Alternatives
Do you smoke regularly?	Frequency not specified	Do you smoke one or more cigarettes per day?
I am rarely free of symptoms	Meaning not clear	I have symptoms most of the time, or I never have symptoms
Do you approve of not having regular X-rays?	Meaning not clear	Do you approve of regular X-rays being cancelled?
Did he sleep normally?	Meaning not clear	Was he asleep for a shorter time than usual?
What type of margarine do you use?	Frequency not specific	What type of margarine do you *usually* use?
How often do you have a blood test?	Frequency not specific	How many blood tests have you had in the last three years?
Have you ever had your AHR measured?	Uses medical jargon	Have you ever had a breathing test to measure your response to inhaled histamine?
Has your child had a red or itchy rash?	Two questions in one sentence	Has your child had a red rash? If yes, was this rash itchy?
Was the workshop too easy or too difficult?	Two questions in one sentence	Rate your experience of the workshop on the 7-point scale below
Do you agree or disagree with the government's policy on health reform?	Two questions in one sentence	Do you agree with the government's policy on health reform?

Table 3.18 shows questions used in an international surveillance of asthma and allergy in which bold type and capitalisation was used to reinforce meaning.

When translating a questionnaire into another language, ask a second person who is fluent in the language to back-translate the questions to ensure that the correct meaning has been retained.

Table 3.18   Questions with special type to emphasise meaning[26]

In the last 12 months, have you had wheezing or whistling in the chest when you **HAD** a cold or flu?	☐₁ No	☐₂ Yes
In the last 12 months, have you had wheezing or whistling in the chest when you **DID NOT HAVE** a cold or flu?	☐₁ No	☐₂ Yes

Presentation and data quality

The visual aspects of the questionnaire are vitally important. The questionnaire is more likely to be completed, and completed accurately, if it is attractive, short and simple. Short questionnaires are likely to attract a better response rate than longer questionnaires.[27] A good questionnaire has a large font, sufficient white space so that the questions are not too dense, numbered questions, clear skip instructions to save time, information of how to answer each question and boxes that are large enough to write in.

Because of their simplicity, tick boxes elicit more accurate responses than asking subjects to circle numbers, put a cross on a line or estimate a percentage or a frequency. These types of responses are also much simpler to code and enter into a database. An example of a user-friendly questionnaire is shown in Table 3.24 at the end of this chapter.

Questions that do not always require a reply should be avoided because they make it impossible to distinguish negative responses from missing data. For example, in Table 3.19, boxes that are not ticked may have been skipped inadvertently or may be negative responses. In addition, there is inconsistent use of the terms 'usually', 'seldom' and 'on average' to elicit information of the frequency of behaviours for which information is required. A better approach would be to have a yes/no option for each question, or to omit the adverbs and use a scale ranging from always to never for each question as shown in Table 3.20.

Table 3.19   Example of inconsistent questions

Tick all of the following that apply to your child:

Usually waves goodbye	☐
Seldom upset when parent leaves	☐
Shows happiness when parent returns	☐
Shy with strangers	☐
Is affectionate, on average	☐

To improve accuracy, it is a good idea to avoid using time responses such as regular, often or occasional, which mean different things to different people, and instead ask whether the event occurred in a variety of frequencies such as:

- ❑ <1/yr
- ❑ 1–6 times/yr
- ❑ 7–12 times/yr
- ❑ >12 times/yr

Other tools, such as the use of filter questions or skips to direct the flow to the next appropriate question, can also increase acceptability and improve data quality.

Remember to always include a thank you at the end of the questionnaire.

Developing scales

It is sometimes useful to collect ordered responses in the form of visual analogue scales (VAS). A commonly used example of a 5-point scale is shown in Table 3.20. Because data collected using these types of scales usually have to be analysed using non-parametric statistical analyses, the use of this type of scale as an outcome measurement often requires a larger sample size than when a normally-distributed, continuous measurement is used. However, scales provide greater statistical power than outcomes based on a smaller number of categories, such as questions which only have 'yes' or 'no' as alternative responses.

Table 3.20   Five-point scale for coded responses to a question
Constant ☐$_1$ Frequent ☐$_2$ Occasional ☐$_3$ Rare ☐$_4$ Never ☐$_5$

In some cases, the usefulness of scales can be improved by recognising that many people are reluctant to use the ends of the scale. For example, it may be better to expand the scale above from five points to seven points by adding points for 'almost never' and 'almost always' before the endpoints 'never' and 'always'. Expanded scales can also increase the responsiveness of questions. If the scale is too short it will not be responsive to measuring subtle within-subject changes in an illness condition or to distinguishing between people with different severity of responses. A way around this is to expand the 5-point scale shown in Table 3.20 to a 9-point Borg score as shown in Table 3.21 with inclusion of mid-points between each of the categories. This increases the responsiveness of the scale and improves its ability to measure smaller changes in symptom severity.

If the pilot study shows that responses are skewed towards one end of the scale or clustered in the centre, then the scale will need to be re-aligned to create a more even range as shown in Table 3.22.

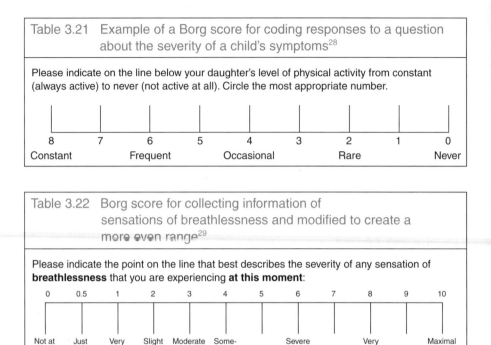

Table 3.21   Example of a Borg score for coding responses to a question about the severity of a child's symptoms[28]

Please indicate on the line below your daughter's level of physical activity from constant (always active) to never (not active at all). Circle the most appropriate number.

8	7	6	5	4	3	2	1	0
Constant		Frequent		Occasional		Rare		Never

Table 3.22   Borg score for collecting information of sensations of breathlessness and modified to create a more even range[29]

Please indicate the point on the line that best describes the severity of any sensation of **breathlessness** that you are experiencing **at this moment**:

0	0.5	1	2	3	4	5	6	7	8	9	10
Not at all	Just notice- able	Very slight	Slight	Moderate	Some- what severe		Severe		Very severe		Maximal

Data collection forms

As with questionnaires, data collection forms are essential for recording study measurements in a standardised and error-free way. For this, the forms need to be practical, clear and easy to use. These attributes are maximised if the form has ample space and non-ambiguous self-coding boxes to ensure accurate data recording. An example of a self-coding data collection form is shown in Table 3.25 at the end of this chapter. Although it is sometimes feasible to avoid the use of coding forms and to enter the data directly into a computer, this is only recommended if security of the data file is absolutely guaranteed. For most research situations, it is much safer to have a hard copy of the results that can be used for documentation, for back-up in case of file loss or computer failure, and for making checks on the quality of data entry.

For maintaining quality control and for checking errors, the identity of the observer should also be recorded on the data collection forms. When information from the data collection forms is merged with questionnaire information or other electronic information into a master database, at least two matching fields must be used in order to avoid matching errors when identification numbers are occasionally transposed, missing or inaccurate.

Coding

Questionnaires and data collection forms must be designed to minimise any measurement error and to make the data easy to collect, process and analyse. For this, it is important to design forms that minimise the potential for data recording errors, which increase bias, and that minimise the number of missing data items, which reduce statistical power, especially in longitudinal studies.

It is sensible to check the questionnaires for completeness of all replies at the time of collection and to follow up missing items as soon as possible in order to increase the efficiency of the study and the generalisability of the results. By ensuring that all questions are self-coding, the time-consuming task of manually coding answers can be largely avoided. These procedures will reduce the time and costs of data coding, data entry and data checking/correcting procedures, and will maximise the statistical power needed to test the study hypotheses.

Pilot studies

Once a draft of a questionnaire has been peer-reviewed to ensure that it has good face validity, it must be pre-tested on a small group of volunteers who are as similar as possible to the target population in whom the questionnaire will be used. The steps that are used in this type of pilot study are shown in Table 3.23. Before a questionnaire is finalised, a number of small pilot studies or an ongoing pilot study may be required so that all problems are identified and the questionnaire can be amended.[30] Data collection forms should also be subjected to a pilot study to ensure that they are complete and function well in practice.

Table 3.23   Pilot study procedures to improve internal validity of a questionnaire

- administer the questionnaire to pilot subjects in exactly the same way as it will be administered in the main study
- ask the subjects for feedback to identify ambiguities and difficult questions
- record the time taken to complete the questionnaire and decide whether it is reasonable
- discard all unnecessary, difficult or ambiguous questions
- assess whether each question gives an adequate range of responses
- establish that replies can be interpreted in terms of the information that is required
- check that all questions are answered
- re-word or re-scale any questions that are not answered as expected
- shorten, revise and, if possible, pilot again

Repeatability and validation

To determine the accuracy of the information collected by the questionnaire, all items will need to be tested for repeatability and to be validated. The methods for measuring repeatability, which involve administering the questionnaire to the same subjects on two occasions, are described in Chapter 7. The methods for establishing various aspects of validity are varied and are described earlier in this chapter.

Internal consistency

The internal consistency of a questionnaire, or a subsection of a questionnaire, is a measure of the extent to which the items provide consistent information. In some situations, factor analysis can be used to determine which questions are useful, which questions are measuring the same or different aspects of health, and which questions are redundant. When developing a score, the weights that need to be applied to each item can be established using factor analysis or logistic regression to ensure that each item contributes appropriately to the total score.

Cronbach's alpha can be used to assess the degree of correlation between items. For example, if a group of twelve questions is used to measure different aspects of stress, then the responses should be highly correlated with one another. As such, Cronbach's alpha provides information that is complementary to that gained by factor analysis and is usually most informative in the development of questionnaires in which a series of scales are used to rate conditions. Unlike repeatability, but in common with factor analysis, Cronbach's alpha can be calculated from a single administration of the questionnaire.

As with all correlation coefficients, Cronbach's alpha has a value between zero and one. If questions are omitted and Cronbach's alpha increases, then the set of questions becomes more reliable for measuring the health trait of interest. However, a Cronbach's alpha value that is too high suggests that some items are giving identical information to other items and could be omitted. Making judgments about including or excluding items by assessing Cronbach's alpha can be difficult because this value increases with an increasing number of items. To improve validity, it is important to achieve a balanced judgment between clinical experience, the interpretation of the data that each question will collect, the repeatability statistics and the exact purpose of the questionnaire.

Table 3.24	Self-coding questions used in a process evaluation of successful grant applications

1. Study design? (tick one)

RCT □1
Non-randomised clinical trial □2
Cohort study □3
Case control study □4
Cross-sectional study □5
Ecological study □6
Qualitative study □7
Other (please specify) _____ □8

2. Status of project?

If not begun, please go to Question 5

Not yet begun □1
Abandoned or suspended □2
In progress □3
Completed □4

3. Number of journal articles from this project?

Published □□
Submitted □□
In progress □□

4. Did this study enable you to obtain external funding from:

Industry □1 No □2 Yes
An external funding body □1 No □2 Yes
Commonwealth or State government □1 No □2 Yes
Donated funds □1 No □2 Yes
Other (please state) _____ □1 No □2 Yes

5. Please rate your experience with each of the following:

i. Amount received   Very satisfied □1   Satisfied □2   Dissatisfied □3
ii. Guidelines   Very satisfied □1   Satisfied □2   Dissatisfied □3
iii. Feedback from committee   Very satisfied □1   Satisfied □2   Dissatisfied □3

Thank you for your assistance

Health science research

Table 3.25   Data recording sheet

ATOPY RECORDING SHEET

Project number	☐ ☐ ☐ ☐
Subject number	☐ ☐ ☐ ☐
Date (ddmmyy)	☐ ☐ ☐ ☐ ☐ ☐

CHILD'S NAME Surname _____ First name _____

Height	☐ ☐ ☐.☐ cms
Weight	☐ ☐.☐ kg
Age	☐ ☐ years
Gender	☐ Male ☐ Female

SKIN TESTS

Tester ID ☐☐   Reader ID ☐☐

Antigen	10 minutes		15 minutes	
	Diameters of skin wheal (mm x mm)	Mean (mm)	Diameters of skin wheal (mm x mm)	Mean (mm)
Control	☐☐ x ☐☐	☐☐	☐☐ x ☐☐	☐☐
Histamine	☐☐ x ☐☐	☐☐	☐☐ x ☐☐	☐☐
Rye grass pollen	☐☐ x ☐☐	☐☐	☐☐ x ☐☐	☐☐
House-dust mite	☐☐ x ☐☐	☐☐	☐☐ x ☐☐	☐☐
Alternaria mould	☐☐ x ☐☐	☐☐	☐☐ x ☐☐	☐☐
Cat	☐☐ x ☐☐	☐☐	☐☐ x ☐☐	☐☐

OTHER TESTS UNDERTAKEN

Urinary cotinine	☐1 No	☐2 Yes
Repeat skin tests	☐1 No	☐2 Yes
Repeat lung function	☐1 No	☐2 Yes
Parental skin tests	☐1 No	☐2 Yes

4
<u>4</u>

CALCULATING THE SAMPLE SIZE

Section 1—Sample size calculations
Section 2—Interim analyses and stopping rules

Section 1—Sample size calculations

The objectives of this section are to understand:
- the concept of statistical power and clinical importance;
- how to estimate an effect size;
- how to calculate the minimum sample size required for different outcome measurements;
- how to increase statistical power if the number of cases available is limited;
- valid uses of internal pilot studies; and
- how to adjust sample size when multivariate analyses are being used.

Clinical importance and statistical significance

Sample size is one of the most critical issues when designing a research study because the size of the sample affects all aspects of conducting the study and interpreting the results. A research study needs to be large enough to ensure the generalisability and the accuracy of the results, but small enough so that the study question can be answered within the research resources that are available.

The issues to be considered when calculating sample size are shown in Table 4.1. Calculating sample size is a balancing act in which many factors need to be taken into account. These include a difference in the outcome measurements between the study groups that will be considered clinically important, the variability around the measurements that is expected, the resources available and the precision that is required around the result. These factors must be balanced with consideration of the ethics of studying too many or too few subjects.

Table 4.1 Issues in sample size calculations
• Clinical importance—effect size
• Variability—spread of the measurements
• Resource availability—efficiency
• Subject availability—feasibility of recruitment
• Statistical power—precision
• Ethics—balancing sample size against burden to subjects

Sample size is a judgmental issue because a clinically important difference between the study groups may not be statistically significant if the sample size is small, but a small difference between study groups that is clinically meaningless will be statistically significant if the sample size is large enough. Thus, an *oversized study* is one that has the power to show that a small difference without clinical importance is statistically significant. This type of study will waste research resources and may be unethical in its unnecessary enrolment of large numbers of subjects to undergo testing. Conversely, an *undersized study* is one that does not have the power to show that a clinically important difference between groups is statistically significant. This may also be unethical if subjects are studied unnecessarily because the study hypothesis cannot be tested. The essential differences between oversized and undersized studies are shown in Table 4.2.

There are numerous examples of results being reported from small studies that are later overturned by trials with a larger sample size.[1] Although undersized clinical trials are reported in the literature, it is clear that many have inadequate power to detect even moderate treatment effects and have a significant chance of reporting false negative results.[2] Although there are some benefits from conducting a small clinical trial, it must be recognised at all stages of the design and conduct of the trial that no questions about efficacy can be answered, and this should be made clear to the subjects who are being enrolled in the study. In most situations, it is better to abandon a study rather than waste resources on a study with a clearly inadequate sample size.

Before beginning any sample size calculations, a decision first needs to be made about the *power* and *significance* that is required for the study.

Table 4.2   Problems that occur if the sample size is too small or large
If the sample is too small (undersized) • type I or type II errors may occur, with a type II error being more likely • the power will be inadequate to show that a clinically important difference is significant • the estimate of effect will be imprecise • a smaller difference between groups than originally anticipated will fail to reach statistical significance • the study may be unethical because the aims cannot be fulfilled If the sample is too large (oversized) • a small difference that is not clinically important will be statistically significant (type I error) • research resources will be wasted • inaccuracies may result because data quality is difficult to maintain • a high response rate may be difficult to achieve • it may be unethical to study more subjects than are needed

Power and probability

The power and probability of a study are essential considerations to ensure that the results are not prone to type I and type II errors. The characteristics of these two types of errors are shown in Table 4.3.

The power of a study is the chance of finding a statistically significant difference when in fact there is one, or of rejecting the null hypothesis. A *type II error* occurs when the null hypothesis is accepted in error, or, put another way, when a false negative result is found. Thus, power is expressed as 1–b, where b is the chance of a type II error occurring. When the b level is 0.1 or 10 per cent, the power of the study is then 0.9 or 90 per cent. In practice, the b level is usually set at 0.2, or 20 per cent, and the power is then 1–b or 0.8 or 80 per cent. A type II error, which occurs when there is a clinically important difference between two groups that does not reach statistical significance, usually arises because the sample size is too small.

The *probability*, or the 'a' level, is the level at which a difference is regarded as statistically significant. As the probability level decreases, the statistical significance of a result increases. In describing the probability level, 5 per cent and 0.05 mean the same thing and sometimes are confusingly described as 95 per cent or 0.95. In most studies, the a rate is set at 0.05, or 5 per cent. An a error, or *type I error*, occurs when a clinical difference between groups does not actually exist but a statistical association is found or, put another way, when the null hypothesis is erroneously rejected. Type I errors usually arise when there is sampling bias or, less commonly, when the sample size is very large or very small.

Table 4.3 Type I and type II errors

Type I errors
- a statistically significant difference is found although the magnitude of the difference is not clinically important
- the finding of a difference between groups when one does not exist
- the erroneous rejection of the null hypothesis

Type II errors
- a clinically important difference between two groups that does not reach statistical significance
- the failure to find a difference between two groups when one exists
- the erroneous acceptance of the null hypothesis

The consequences of type I and type II errors are very different. If a study is designed to test whether a new treatment is more effective than an existing treatment, then the null hypothesis would be that there is no difference between the two treatments. If the study design results in a type I error, then the null hypothesis will be erroneously rejected and the new treatment will be judged to be better than the existing treatment. In situations where the new treatment is more expensive or has more severe side effects, this will impose an unnecessary burden on patients. On the other hand, if the study design results in a type II error, then the new treatment may be judged as being no better than the existing treatment even though it has some benefits. In this situation, many patients may be denied the new treatment because it will be judged as a more expensive option with no apparent advantages.

Calculating sample size

An adequate sample size ensures a high chance of finding that a clinically important difference between two groups is statistically significant, and thus minimises the chance of finding type I or type II errors. However, the final choice of sample size is always a delicate balance between the expected variance in the measurements, the availability of prospective subjects and the expected rates of non-compliance or drop-outs, and the feasibility of collecting the data. In essence, sample size calculations are a rough estimate of the minimum number of subjects needed in a study. The limitations of a sample size estimated before the study commences are shown in Table 4.4.

Table 4.4	Sample size calculations do not make allowance for the following situations:
<ul><li>the variability in the measurements being larger than expected</li><li>subjects who drop out</li><li>subjects who fail to attend or do not comply with the intervention</li><li>having to screen subjects who do not fulfil the eligibility criteria</li><li>subjects with missing data</li><li>providing the power to conduct subgroup analyses</li></ul>	

If there is more than one outcome variable, the sample size is usually calculated for the primary outcome on which the main hypothesis is based, but this rarely provides sufficient power to test the secondary hypotheses, to conduct multivariate analyses or to explore interactions. In intervention trials, a larger sample size will be required for analyses based on intention-to-treat principles than for analyses based on compliance with the intervention. In most intervention studies, it is accepted that compliance rates of over 80 per cent are difficult to achieve. However, if 25 per cent of subjects are non-compliant, then the sample size will need to be much larger and may need to be doubled in order to maintain the statistical power to demonstrate a significant effect.

In calculating sample size, the benefits of conducting a study that is too large need to be balanced against the problems that occur if the study is too small. The problems that can occur if the sample size is too large or too small were shown in Table 4.2. One of the main disadvantages of small studies is that the estimates of effect are imprecise, that is they have a large standard error and therefore large confidence intervals around the result. This means that the outcome, such as a mean value or an odds ratio, will not be precise enough for meaningful interpretation. As such, the result may be ambiguous, for example a confidence interval of 0.6–1.6 around an odds ratio does not establish whether an intervention has a protective or positive effect.

Subgroup analyses

When analysing the results of a research study, it is common to examine the main study hypothesis and then go on to examine whether the effects are larger or smaller in various subgroups, such as males and females or younger and older patients. However, sample size calculations only provide sufficient statistical power to test the main hypotheses and need to be multiplied by the number of levels in the subgroups in order to provide this additional power. For example, to test for associations in males and females separately the sample size would have to be doubled if there is fairly even recruitment of male and female subjects, or may need to be increased even further if one gender is more likely to be recruited.

Although computer packages are available for calculating sample sizes for various applications, the simplest method is to consult a table. Because sample size calculations are only ever a rough estimate of the minimum sample size, computer programs sometimes confer a false impression of accuracy. Tables are also useful for planning meetings when computer software may not be available.

Categorical outcome variables

The number of subjects needed for comparing the prevalence of an outcome in two study groups is shown in Table 4.5. To use the table, the prevalence of the outcome in the study and control groups has to be estimated and the size of the difference in prevalence between groups that would be regarded as clinically important or of public health significance has to be nominated. The larger the difference between the rates, the smaller the sample size required in each group.

Table 4.5 Approximate sample size needed in each group to detect a significant difference in prevalence rates between two populations for a power of 80 per cent and a significance of 5 per cent

Smaller rate	Difference in rates (p_1-p_2)						
	5%	10%	15%	20%	30%	40%	50%
5%	480	160	90	60	35	25	20
10%	730	220	115	80	40	25	20
20%	1140	320	150	100	45	30	20
30%	1420	380	180	110	50	30	20
40%	1570	410	190	110	50	30	20
50%	1610	410	190	110	50	30	–

This method of estimating sample size applies to analyses that are conducted using chi-square tests or McNemar's test for paired proportions.

However, they do not apply to conditions with a prevalence or incidence of less than 5 per cent for which more complex methods based on a Poisson distribution are needed. When using Table 4.5, the sample size for prevalence rates higher than 50 per cent can be estimated by using 100 per cent minus the prevalence rate on each axis of the table, for example for 80 per cent use 100 per cent–80 per cent, or 20 per cent. An example of a sample size calculation using Table 4.5, is shown in Example 4.1.

Figure 4.1

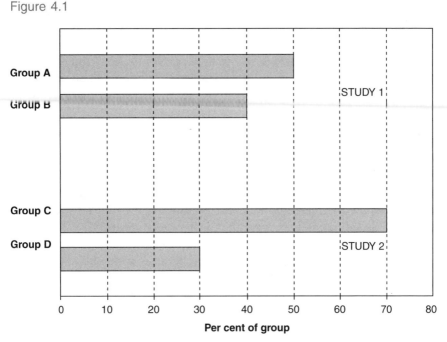

Prevalence rates of a primary outcome in two groups in two different studies (1 and 2).

Example 4.1   Sample size calculations for categorical data

For example, if the sample size that is required to show that two prevalence rates of 40% and 50% as shown in Study 1 in Figure 4.1 needs to be estimated, then
Difference in rates = 50%–40% = 10%
Smaller rate = 40%
Minimum sample size required = 410 in each group
If the sample size that is required to show that two prevalence rates of 30% and 70% as shown in Study 2 in Figure 4.1 needs to be estimated, then
Difference in rates = 70%–30% = 40%
Smaller rate = 30%
Minimum sample size required = 30 in each group

Examples for describing sample size calculations in studies with categorical outcome variables are shown in Table 4.13 later in this chapter.

Confidence intervals around prevalence estimates

The larger a sample size, the smaller that the confidence interval around the estimate of prevalence will be. The relationship between sample size and 95 per cent confidence intervals is shown in Figure 4.2. For the same estimate of prevalence, the confidence interval is very wide for a small sample size of ten subjects but quite small for a sample size of 1000 subjects.

Figure 4.2   Influence of sample size on confidence intervals

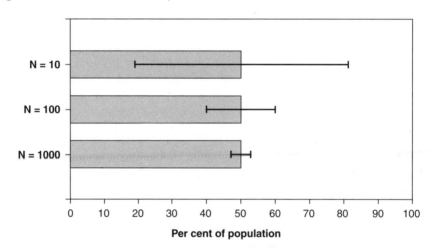

Prevalence rate and confidence intervals showing how the width of the confidence interval, that is the precision of the estimate, decreases with increasing sample size.

In Figure 4.3, it can be seen that if 32 subjects are enrolled in each group, the difference between an outcome of 25 per cent in one group and 50 per cent in the other is not statistically significant as shown by the confidence intervals that overlap. However, if the number of subjects in each group is doubled to 64, then the confidence intervals are reduced to no overlap, which is consistent with a P value of less than 0.01.

One method for estimating sample size in a study designed to measure prevalence in a single group is to nominate the level of precision that is required around the prevalence estimate and then to calculate the sample size needed to attain this. Table 4.6 shows the sample size required to calculate prevalence for each specified width of the 95 per cent confidence interval. Again, the row for a prevalence rate of 5 per cent also applies to a prevalence rate of 100 per cent–5 per cent, or 95 per cent.

Table 4.6	Approximate sample size required to calculate a prevalence rate with the precision shown								
	Width of 95% confidence interval (precision)								
Prevalence	1%	1.5%	2%	2.5%	3%	4%	5%	10%	15%
5%	2000	800	460	290	200	110	70	35	–
10%	3400	1550	870	550	380	220	140	40	20
15%	5000	2200	1200	780	550	300	200	50	20
20%	6200	2700	1500	1000	700	400	250	60	25
25%	8000	3200	1800	1150	800	450	290	70	32

Thus, if the prevalence of the outcome in a study is estimated to be 15 per cent, a sample size of 300 will be required to produce a confidence interval of 4 per cent, 550 for a confidence interval of 3 per cent and 1200 for a confidence interval of 2 per cent. An example of how confidence intervals and sample size impact on the interpretation of differences in prevalence rates is shown in Figure 4.3 and Example 4.2.

Figure 4.3   Interpretation of confidence intervals

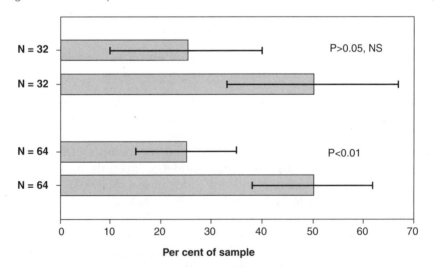

Similar prevalence rates in two studies with different sample sizes showing how the confidence intervals no longer overlap and the difference between the groups becomes significant when the sample size is increased.

Figure 4.4

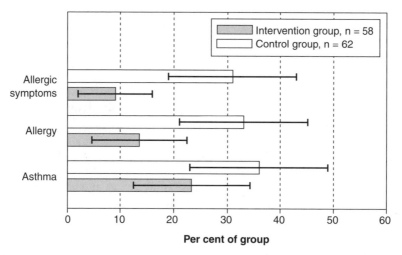

Prevalence of three outcomes variables in a control and intervention group in a randomised controlled trial to measure the effectiveness of an intervention in preventing the onset of asthma in early childhood.[3]

Example 4.2   Possible type II error

Figure 4.4 shows the results from a study in which various symptoms of asthma and allergy were measured in an intervention study.[3] In this study, there were 58 subjects in the intervention group (shaded bars) and 62 subjects in the control group (white bars). The study had sufficient power to show that the prevalence of allergic symptoms and reactions to specific allergens were different between the study groups but was under-powered to show that a difference of 11% in the prevalence of asthma between groups was statistically significant. From Table 4.5, a sample size of 320 subjects in each group would have been needed to show that a 10% difference in the prevalence of asthma between groups was significantly different.

Rare events

It can be difficult to estimate a required sample size when the main outcome of interest is rare. This can occur in studies such as surgical trials when a new procedure is being investigated and the aim of the study is to confirm that serious adverse outcomes do not occur. It is important to remember that a study in which an event does not occur does not necessarily mean that the intervention or procedure has no risk. In this type of study, the upper limit of risk can be computed as 3 divided by the sample size $(3/n)$.[4]

For estimating sample size for studies designed to measure rare events, an upper limit of risk needs to be nominated, and then by substitution the sample size can be calculated. If the upper limit of risk is one in ten patients, that is 10 per cent or a proportion of 0.1, then the sample size required to confirm that the risk of an event is less than 10 per cent is 3/0.1, or 30 subjects. If the upper limit of risk is much lower at 1 per cent, or 0.01, then a sample size of 3/0.01, or 300 subjects, is required to confirm that the intervention has an acceptably low rate of adverse events.

Effect of compliance on sample size

In clinical trials, the power of the study to show a difference between the study groups is reduced if some of the subjects do not comply with the intervention. If the proportion of non-compliers in the active intervention arm, or the proportion of non-compliers plus subjects who change to the standard treatment arm, is NC then the sample size has to be increased by a factor size of 1 divided by $(1-NC)^2$. The inflation factors for various estimates of non-compliance are shown in Table 4.7. If the rate of non-compliance is as high as 30 per cent, then the sample size of the intervention group may need to be increased by 100 per cent, that is doubled. For this reason, methods that can be used to increase and maintain compliance in the active intervention arm are usually cost-effective because they maintain the statistical power of a study to demonstrate a clinically important effect.

Table 4.7   Size of inflation factor to increase sample size if a proportion of subjects in the active intervention arm are non-compliant or change to the standard treatment arm

Rate non-compliance in active intervention group (%)	Approximate inflation factor for sample size calculation (%)
10	20
15	40
20	56
30	100

Another method of maintaining power is to have a run-in period in clinical trials. During the run-in period, baseline measurements can be monitored and compliance with the medication regime and with completing the outcome forms can be assessed. Eliminating non-compliant subjects during the run-in phase and prior to randomisation is an effective method of maintaining the power of the study and may be appropriate in studies that are designed to measure efficacy. However this approach limits the generalisability of the study and is not appropriate in studies of effectiveness.

Continuous outcome variables

The sample size that is needed for analyses of continuous outcome variables is shown in Table 4.8.[5] This table can be used for estimating sample size for analyses that require an unpaired two-tailed t-test to compare the mean values in two independent groups, or that require a paired t-test to assess the significance of the mean change from baseline in a single sample.

To use Table 4.8, a decision needs to be made about the study outcome that is of greatest importance to the study aims, that is the primary outcome variable. The next step is to estimate the expected mean and standard deviation of this measurement in the reference or control group. From this, a nominated *effect size*, that is the size of the minimum difference between cases and controls, or between study groups, that would be regarded as clinically important can be estimated. The effect size, which is expressed in units of the standard deviation, is sometimes called the *minimal clinically important difference*.

Figure 4.5

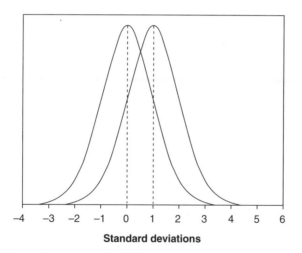

Standard deviations

Normal distribution of a continuously distributed measurement in two groups of subjects showing that the means are separated by a distance, or effect size, of one standard deviation.

Example 4.3   Calculation of effect size

Figure 4.5 shows the distribution of a continuous outcome variable in two groups who differ by an effect size of one standard deviation, shown by the distance between the two dotted vertical lines. For this effect size, 18–24 subjects per group would be required to demonstrate a significant difference.

Table 4.8   Sample size for unpaired and paired means (a rate = 0.05)
The sample size shown is the number of subjects per group for unpaired data and the total number of subjects for paired data

Effect size[a]	Unpaired data		Paired data[b]	
	power=80%	power=90%	power=80%	power=90%
0.25	255	375	128	190
0.35	130	175	66	88
0.5	64	95	34	50
0.75	30	45	16	24
1.0	18	24	10	14
1.25	12	16	7	9
1.5	9	12	–	8
2.0	6	7	–	–

[a] in units of standard deviations
[b] for paired data, the standard deviation of the difference is required

For paired data, effect size is the distance of the mean from zero, estimated in units of the standard deviation of the paired differences. Thus a smaller sample size is needed because there is no variation around the zero value. However, if a change from baseline is being compared in two independent groups, such as cases and controls, then the problem becomes a two-sample t-test again in which the outcome being considered in each group is change from baseline. In this case, the column for unpaired data is used and the estimate of effect size is based on the mean and standard deviation of the differences from baseline in the control group.

Non-parametric outcome measurements

If the outcome is not normally distributed and non-parametric statistics will be used, then the sample size can also be estimated using Table 4.8. Since the effect size cannot be based on a standard deviation, a nominal effect size has to be proposed. For safety, the higher power value of 90 per cent needs to be used and at least 10 per cent should also be added to the sample size.

There is only a modest saving in the required sample size if the outcome has more than two categories compared to a binary outcome.[6] Therefore, sample size for data collected using three-, five- or seven-point Borg scores or Likert scales can be estimated from Table 4.5. In this case, the sample size is calculated as the power to detect a difference in the number of subjects above or below a nominated point on the scale.

Balancing the number of cases and controls

When an illness is rare and only a small number of potential subjects are available, statistical power can be increased by enrolling a greater number of control subjects; that is, two or more controls for every case. Unbalanced studies are also sometimes used to test the efficacy of new treatments when more information is required about the new treatment than about current best practice. The approach of using unbalanced groups is also useful if the number of subjects who receive a treatment or intervention has to be limited because it is expensive. Table 4.9 shows the trade-off between an increase in power and the extra number of subjects who need to be studied. In studies in which unbalanced groups are used, there is a decreasing efficiency as the degree of unbalance increases, with little gain in extending the ratio of cases to controls beyond 1:3 or 1:4.

Table 4.9 'Trade-off' effect by increasing the number of control subjects			
Ratio of cases: controls	Number of cases: controls	Total subjects	Sample size required if numbers equal
1:1	25:25	50	50
1:2	25:50	75	66
1:3	25:75	100	76
1:4	25:100	125	80
1:5	25:125	150	84
1:10	25:250	275	90

Odds ratio and relative risk

The sample size that is required to measure a statistically significant odds ratio or relative risk is shown in Table 4.10 with an example of how to describe the sample size calculation shown in Table 4.13 at the end of this section. If logistic regression is used, a general rule of thumb is to add at least 10 per cent to the sample size for each variable in the model. If stratification by confounders is being used, then the sample size requirements shown in Table 4.10 will apply to each strata in the analyses.

The sample size for an odds ratio of r is the same as the sample size for an odds ratio of $1/r$, for example the sample size for an odds ratio of 2 is the same as for an odds ratio of 0.5. However, in epidemiological studies in which the measure of exposure is poor, then the sample size needs to be increased accordingly. The sample size may need to be doubled if the correlation between the measurement and the true exposure is less than 0.8, and tripled for a correlation less than 0.6.[7]

Table 4.10 can also be used as an approximation for calculating the sample size for measuring odds ratios in matched case-control studies in which the effects of confounders are controlled in the study design. However, unnecessary matching of subjects results in a loss of efficiency and therefore the need for a larger sample size. A sample size that is up to 50 per cent higher may be required in matched studies if the outcome is rare (less than 10 per cent) or if the matching variable is a weak or uncertain risk factor for the disease being investigated.[8]

Table 4.10 Approximate total minimum sample size for detecting a statistically significant odds ratio in an unmatched case-control study given the proportion of controls who are exposed to the factor of interest (power=80%, significance=0.05)

Proportion of controls exposed	Odds ratio					
	1.5	2.0	2.5	3.0	4.0	5.0
0.1	960	310	170	120	70	50
0.2	570	190	110	70	50	40
0.3	450	160	90	65	45	35
0.4	410	150	90	65	45	35
0.5	410	150	90	65	45	35

Correlation coefficients

The sample size required to find a significant association between two continuous measurements is shown in Table 4.11. Because a correlation coefficient is significant if it is statistically different from zero, a P value of less than 0.05 does not always mean that one variable explains a clinically important proportion of the variability in the other variable.

Table 4.11 Total sample size for detecting a correlation coefficient which is statistically significant from zero at the $P<0.05$ level

Correlation	$\alpha=0.05$ power=80%	$\alpha=0.05$ power=90%
0.1	780	1050
0.2	200	260
0.3	85	120
0.4	50	60
0.5	30	40
0.6	20	25
0.7	15	20

Repeatability and agreement

Very little attention has been given to the power of studies used to calculate repeatability and agreement although, in common with all studies, precision is an important concept.

The methods of expressing repeatability and agreement between observers and between methods are varied with no formal methods for calculating minimum sample size requirements. Obviously, a larger sample size will provide a more precise estimate of both the measurement error and the intraclass correlation coefficient (ICC). The measurement error is an absolute estimate of how much reliance can be placed on a measurement whereas the ICC is a relative estimate of the proportion of variance that can be attributed to 'true' differences between the subjects (Chapter 7). If repeatability is being measured, increased precision can be obtained by increasing the sample size or by increasing the number of measurements taken from each subject, which is useful in situations in which the number of subjects is limited.

For estimating repeatability from two measurements, a sample size of 30 subjects is the bare minimum, 50 subjects is adequate and 100 subjects gives good precision. A sample size larger than 100 subjects is usually unnecessary. For estimating agreement between two continuously distributed measurements, a sample size of 100 gives good precision and above this, the efficiency in reducing the standard error rapidly declines.[9] However, larger numbers are often need for categorical data, such as data collected by questionnaires.

Both the size of the ICC expected and the number of measurements taken from each subject will influence the precision with which estimates of repeatability are calculated. Thus, a sample size requirement for a study in which three repeated measures are collected may be a minimum of 50 subjects but for only two repeated measures, the sample size will need to be larger for the same ICC value. Also, a rule of thumb is that a larger number is needed for the same precision in an ICC value calculated from two-way analysis of variance (ANOVA) than for an ICC value calculated from one-way ANOVA, although there are no simple methods to calculate the difference.

For estimates of kappa, which is a measure of repeatability of categorical data, a minimum sample size of $2 \times$ (number of categories)^2 is required so that for five categories the estimated minimum sample size would be 50 subjects.[10] In practice, this number may be too small and, as for ICC, a sample size of over 100 subjects with duplicate measurements is usually needed to estimate kappa with precision. The sample size required also depends on the prevalence of the outcome, with factors that have a low prevalence requiring a larger sample size than factors that occur commonly.

Sensitivity and specificity

There are no formal tables for calculating the number of subjects needed to measure the sensitivity and specificity of an instrument. However, these two statistics are merely proportions and the confidence interval around them is calculated in exactly the same way as a confidence interval around any proportion. The sample size required to obtain a confidence interval of a certain width can be estimated separately for the expected sensitivity and specificity statistics using Table 4.6. The sample sizes for calculating sensitivity and specificity are then added together to obtain the total sample size requirement.

Analysis of variance

It is possible to estimate sample size when a one-way analysis of variance (ANOVA) will be used to analyse the data, and this can be extended to a two-way ANOVA by estimating the sample size for each level of the factors included. There are two options—one is to use a nomogram to calculate sample size for up to five groups.[11] The other is to use a method that allows for the expected dispersion of the means between the study groups.[12] The

Effect size	Number of groups	power=80% $\alpha=0.05$	power=90% $\alpha=0.05$
0.1	3	315	415
	4	270	350
	5	240	310
0.2	3	80	105
	4	68	90
	5	60	80
0.3	3	36	48
	4	32	40
	5	28	35
0.4	3	22	28
	4	18	24
	5	16	20
0.5	3	14	18
	4	12	15
	5	12	14

Table 4.12 Sample size requirements, that is number per group, for one-way analysis of variance[13]

approximate adjustment factor is 0.4 for three or four groups and 0.3 for five or six groups. However, if the mean values are dispersed at the ends of the range with none in the middle, an adjustment factor of 0.5 is used.

The sample size is then estimated by calculating the effect size, that is the difference between the lowest and the highest means, in units of the standard deviation, and multiplying this by the adjustment factor, that is:

$$\text{Effect size} = \frac{\text{highest mean} - \text{lowest mean}}{\text{standard deviation}}$$

$$\text{Adjusted effect size} = \text{effect size} \times \text{adjustment factor}$$

The adjusted effect size can then be used to calculate sample size using Table 4.12. In practice, 0.1 to 0.2 is a small effect size, 0.25 to 0.4 is a medium effect size, and effect sizes of 0.5 or more are large.

For repeated measures ANOVA, sample size per group can be estimated by using paired data tables and increasing the estimated sample size. A more precise method is to calculate the sample size as for a standard ANOVA and then decrease the sample size because the repeated measurements help to reduce the variance. To make a final decision, it is a good idea to use both methods and then compare the results. For multivariate analysis variance (MANOVA) specialised methods for calculating sample size based on the number of variables and the number of groups are available.[14]

Multivariate analyses

When no formal sample size methods are available for multivariate applications, estimates for continuous outcome variables or ANOVA can be used and the sample size adjusted according to the number of strata or number of variables in the analysis. Remember that covariates that increase the correlation coefficient between the outcome and the explanatory variable also increase statistical power and therefore result in a smaller sample being required.

For all multivariate analyses, an ad-hoc method to confirm the adequacy of the estimated sample size is to consult published studies that have used similar data analyses and assess whether the sample size has provided adequate precision around the estimates.

A minimum requirement for *logistic regression* is that the subjects must number at least ten times the number of variables.[15] However, this may not provide sufficient precision for estimating the confidence intervals around the odds ratios. Another approach to use Table 4.10 to estimate a sample size for an expected odds ratio, and increase the sample size by at least 10 per cent for every extra variable included in the analysis. Other more detailed and more complicated methods are available in the literature.[16]

Survival analyses

For survival analyses, the power to compare survival in two or more groups is related more to the number of events (e.g. deaths) than to the total sample size, with a very large sample size being needed if the risk of the event occurring is very small. In such studies, power can be increased by increasing the length of follow-up or by increasing the number of subjects. For this, formal sample size calculation tables are available in specialised texts.[17]

Describing sample size calculations

Table 4.13   Describing sample size calculations
Comparing prevalence rates
1. The sample size has been calculated with the aim of being able to demonstrate that the prevalence of the outcome is 50% lower in the intervention group, that is it will be reduced from 60% to 30%. For a power of 90% and a significance level of 0.05, a minimum number of 118 children will be needed in each group. To allow for a 20% drop-out rate in the first three years, at least 150 children will be enrolled in each group. 2. We expect that the prevalence of the outcome will be approximately 10% in the reference group. Therefore, a minimum of 220 subjects will be enrolled in each of the two study groups. This sample size will give an 80% power of detecting a difference in prevalence between the two groups of 10% with significance at the $P<0.05$ level.
Single prevalence rates
The prevalence of this condition in the community is expected to be in the order of 10%–15%. Therefore, a sample size of 1200 has been chosen with the aim of being able to estimate the prevalence with a 95% confidence interval of ± 2%.
Continuous outcome variables
1. This sample size will allow us to detect a significant difference if the mean of the outcome variable for the cases is at least 1 standard deviation higher than the mean value for the control group (power=80%, significance=0.05). 2. A total number of 50 subjects will allow us to demonstrate that a mean within-subject change from baseline of 0.5 standard deviations is significant at the 0.05 level with a power of 90%.

Cont'd

Table 4.13 Cont'd   Describing sample size calculations

3. A total of 64 subjects will be required in each group in order to detect a difference between groups of 0.5 standard deviations in height. However, only 50 cases are expected to be available in the next year. Therefore, two control subjects will be enrolled for each case in order to maintain statistical power. This will give a total study sample of 150 subjects.
Odds ratios
Assuming that 30% of the controls will be exposed to (the study factor of interest), a sample size of 180 subjects, that is 90 cases and 90 controls, will be needed. This will allow us to detect an odds ratio of 2.5 with statistical significance (power=80%, significance=95%). This magnitude of odds ratio represents a clinically important increase of risk of illness in the presence of (outcome of interest).
Analysis of variance
We are comparing the outcome of interest between four study groups. An effect size of one standard deviation between the lowest and highest groups is expected with the mean values of each of the other two groups falling within this. The adjustment factor is therefore calculated to be 0.37 and the minimum number of subjects required in each group will be 40. Thus, for a power of 90% and a significance level of 0.05, we will require a minimum sample size of 160 subjects.

Section 2—Interim analyses and stopping rules

The objectives of this section are to understand:
- when interim analyses are justified;
- when to make the decision to stop a clinical trial; and
- the problems caused by stopping a study prematurely.

Interim analyses

Any analyses that are undertaken before all of the subjects have been recruited and the study is completed are called interim analyses. These types of analysis can play a useful part in the management of clinical trials. Interim analyses can be used to decide whether to continue a trial to compare the efficacy of two treatments as it was planned, or whether to only continue the study of the 'superior' treatment group. Interim analyses are also useful for re-assessing the adequacy of the planned sample size. However, the number of interim analyses must be planned, must be limited and must be carried out under strictly controlled conditions so that the scientific integrity of the study is maintained and unbiased evidence about the benefits of a new treatment or intervention is collected.

If interim analyses are undertaken regularly, they increase the chance of finding a false positive result. To avoid this, it is essential to plan the number and the timing of all interim analyses, as far as possible, in the study design stage of the study before the data are collected.[18] Also, when unplanned interim analyses are performed, the significance level that is used must be altered. Thus, if ten annual interim analyses are planned, a simple strategy is to use a significance level of $P<0.01$ or $P<0.005$ for each analysis rather than $P<0.05$.[19] Another suggestion is to use a nominal significance level of P<0.001 in unplanned interim analyses and then to redesign the study so that any further interim analyses are only conducted when planned.[20]

To avoid increasing or creating bias, the interim analyses should be undertaken by members of a data monitoring committee who have no active involvement in the study. Whenever interim analyses are conducted, it is essential that the results are not released to the research team who are responsible for collecting the data because this information may increase observer bias, and selection bias if recruitment is continuing.

Glossary

Term	Meaning
Interim analysis	An analysis that is conducted before all of the subjects have been enrolled and have completed the study
Type I and II errors	False positive and false negative research results (see Table 4.3)
Statistical power	The ability of the study to show that a clinically important result is statistically significant

Internal pilot studies

Internal pilot studies can be used to confirm sample size calculations. A *priori* sample size calculations underestimate the sample size required when the variance in the reference group is wider than expected. This commonly occurs when the variance has been estimated in previous studies that have a small sample size or different inclusion criteria. One way to confirm that the sample size is adequate is to conduct an internal pilot study. This involves analysing the data from the first control subjects enrolled into a study in order to recalculate the variance in this reference group, and then using this information to recalculate the required sample size. As with all interim analyses, the researchers collecting the data must remain blinded to the results. It is also crucial that the internal pilot study data are not used to prematurely test the study hypotheses.

Internal pilot studies are different from classical pilot studies. Classical pilot studies are small studies that are conducted prior to the commencement of a research study with the express purpose of ensuring that the recruitment procedures are practical, the evaluation tools are appropriate, and the protocol does not need to be changed once the study is underway (Chapter 2). The data from pilot studies are not included with the study data when the results are analysed because they are not collected using the same standardised methods as the study data. In contrast, the data used in an internal pilot study are part of the study data and are therefore included in final analyses.

Internal pilot studies have the advantage that they only have a small effect on the α level of the study but, by estimating sample size more accurately, they have a significant effect on both power and efficiency. A major benefit of recalculating sample size at an early stage in a study is that it provides the opportunity to plan to recruit larger numbers of subjects if this is necessary. Because it is also important that only one internal pilot study is undertaken, a judgment of when the internal pilot will be conducted must be made before the study begins. An internal pilot study should be as large as possible with a minimum sample size of twenty subjects.[21, 22] For example, the internal pilot study may be after the first twenty subjects if the total sample size is expected to be 40, but after the first 100 if the expected sample size is 1000.

Safety analyses

In studies designed to test a new treatment or intervention, processes need to be in place to detect adverse effects at an early stage. In addition, if any adverse effects are suspected, then a safety analysis to estimate whether the effects are significantly higher in the new treatment group will be required. Before a safety analysis is conducted, the difference between groups in the frequency of the adverse event that would be considered clinically important has to be nominated. The sample size that would be required to demonstrate that this difference is statistically significant can then be calculated. Once the required sample size has been recruited, a planned safety analysis can be undertaken and the results evaluated by an external monitoring committee. As with internal pilot studies, the researchers who are responsible for collecting the data must be blinded to the results of the safety analysis.

Stopping a study

Ideally, the decision to stop any research study before the planned sample size is reached should be based on both statistical and ethical issues. This decision needs to balance the interests of the subjects who have not yet been recruited with the interests of the study. There have been examples of interim analyses demonstrating harmful effects of a new treatment, such as toxic effects of cancer treatments. The identification of harmful effects leads to the dilemma that although a large sample size is needed to answer questions about efficacy, there will be reluctance to recruit subjects to receive the more toxic treatment,[23] and the more serious the disease is, the more serious the dilemma becomes.[24]

Glossary

Term	Meaning
Stopping rules	Prior decisions made about when recruitment of subjects may be stopped
Observer bias	Distortion of the results because the observers are aware of the study purpose or the results of the interim analyses
External monitoring committee	Committee with no involvement in conducting the study or interpreting the analyses but who are appointed to oversee the scientific validity of the study

Stopping rules

Clinical trials are sometimes stopped prematurely because a statistically significant result is found that indicates that the new treatment is clearly better or clearly worse than the old treatment. Occasionally, a study may also be stopped because a non-significant result has been reached, that is the new treatment appears to be no better or no worse than the old treatment. However, there are examples in the literature of studies being stopped early[25] and subsequent trials then finding very different results.[26] It is not unusual for interim analyses to produce a false positive result and then for the results of further sequential interim analyses to sequentially converge to null. Thus, the significant result at the first interim analysis becomes increasingly less significant as the study progresses. The adverse effects of stopping a study too early are shown in Table 4.14.

Table 4.14   Adverse outcomes of stopping a study too early[27]
• lack of credibility—results from small studies are not convincing • lack of realism—dramatic treatment differences are not convincing • imprecision—wider confidence intervals for the treatment effect • bias—studies are likely to stop on a 'random high' of treatment differences • excessive speed—insufficient time to consider balance of benefits and costs • undue pressure—over-enthusiastic and unreasonable recommendations may follow • mistakes—the risk of a false positive result

If there is a possibility that the study will be stopped on the basis of an interim analysis before the full sample size is recruited, then ideally, the stopping rules should be decided before the study begins. The decision to stop a study should not be taken lightly because a statistically significant effect of treatment on outcome may be found, but the precision of the estimate will be reduced and the 95 per cent confidence intervals will be much wider than expected. Also, a smaller sample size markedly reduces the statistical power to measure treatment effects in specific subgroups or to conduct multivariate analyses.

To avoid a study resulting in a false positive result, the decision to stop should be based on a high level of significance, that is very small P values. Other formal methods, such as adjusting the significance levels for making formal stopping rules can be used.[28] When the decision to stop is not clear, it is best handed over to an external monitoring committee who have all of the internal and external evidence available to them.[29]

Equipoise

Equipoise is a term that is used to describe the uncertainty in the minds of the researchers of the clinical effectiveness of currently used or experimental treatments. Researchers need to be in this situation of equipoise for the commencement or continuation of a clinical trial to be ethical.[30] Ethical considerations are the most important factor to consider when deciding to continue or stop a study. However, it is inevitable that the decision to continue a study will almost always result in statistical benefits because the optimal sample size requirement will be achieved and power will be maintained to conduct subgroup analyses, or to adjust for confounders in the analyses. Continuation of any clinical trial until the planned stopping time will almost always ensure that the results will have better precision and are less likely to produce a false positive or false negative result than a trial that is stopped early.[31, 32]

5

CONDUCTING THE STUDY

Section 1—Project management

The objectives of this section are to understand:
- how to manage a study; and
- how to ensure that high quality data is collected.

Study management

Once the funding for a research study is received, the data collection stages must be properly planned and conducted so that the scientific integrity of the study is maintained throughout. It is not only unethical to conduct a study that is poor science, it is also unethical to produce poor quality data that inevitably lead to poor quality results.

The principal investigators of a study are responsible for ensuring that the data are collected to a high scientific standard, but this can only be achieved with good management practices.[1] Good management not only involves pro-active forward planning but also involves regular meetings of the study team in order to make collaborative decisions about the study progress and the study processes. A collaborative approach between the management and research teams will help to promote strict adherence to the study protocol by staff at all levels of subject recruitment, data collection and data management.

Data quality assurance

Table 5.1 shows the procedures that can be used to ensure quality control when data are being collected either at a single centre, or by different groups at different centres. There are many advantages of putting these procedures in place, including the prevention of problems and errors that reduce the scientific integrity of the data.[2] The process of involving all researchers in the research process is important for empowering research staff to take pride in their work. This in turn will lead to a climate in which research staff enjoy being part of a collaborative team and will also encourage the development of professional skills.

Table 5.1   Procedures to maintain data quality
❑ Conduct pilot studies to test recruitment procedures and study tools
❑ Hold regular meetings, tele-conferences and site visits that involve all of the research staff
❑ Document all protocol variations
❑ Maintain an up-to-date handbook of all procedures and protocols
❑ Train all data collection staff centrally
❑ Only use pre-tested questionnaires and instruments once the study is underway
❑ Rotate staff regularly between locations to ensure standardisation of data collection methods
❑ Undertake continuous monitoring of the data for errors etc.
❑ Check all data for completeness before data entry
❑ Minimise the number of interim and safety analyses
❑ Ensure that data collection staff are blinded to results of any analyses

It is usually the responsibility of the study co-ordinator to compile and maintain an up-to-date study handbook. Table 5.2 shows a list of some of the methods, protocols and policies that should be included in the handbook. The purpose of the handbook is to maintain a document that itemises all of the methods being used in the study, and that catalogues all of the data collection forms. In any research study, this is an invaluable tool. This handbook must be updated regularly so that all changes to the study protocol and the rationale for making the changes are carefully listed. Any deviations from the protocol should also be documented.

An updated copy of the handbook must be readily available to everyone in the research team. The study handbook should also document information of the location and content of the study databases, the dates and details of any errors that are detected and corrections that are made, and any data coding or recoding schedules. A separate file should also be maintained that contains all of the minutes and the actions from the study meetings.

Table 5.2   Study handbook contents
• position and contact details of investigators and all research staff
• aims or hypotheses
• background and rationale for study
• study design

Cont'd

Table 5.2 Cont'd   Study handbook contents

• subject details including inclusion and exclusion criteria
• method details
• randomisation and allocation concealment procedures
• intervention details
• goods and equipment required
• recruitment strategies
• consent forms and information for participants
• data collection instruments
• rationale for including new questions or questionnaires
• policies for managing anticipated problems
• details of withdrawals and procedures for follow-up
• ethics approvals
• budget and details of donations, incentives, etc.
• data management including confidentiality and access issues
• data coding and recoding schedules
• management of adverse effects and details of safety committee
• changes to protocol, including dates and rationale for changes
• dissemination of study outcomes to participants
• planned data analyses and publications

Monitoring committees

All research studies need a hierarchy of committees to oversee the conduct of the study, the handling of the data and the scientific reports from the study. As well as ensuring that adequate resources are available for conducting the study with scientific integrity, the principal investigators will need to make decisions about the responsibilities and composition of these committees prior to any data being collected. In running a study, especially a large or multi-centre study, it is important to hold regular meetings that are attended by the entire research team, including the researchers who are responsible for collecting the data and the data managers. In addition, closed management meetings to make decisions about protocol details, financial matters and other sensitive issues will also be needed.

The level of responsibility of different committees will vary considerably. Internal committees may only include the investigators and their research staff. However, the membership of an external committee may include a number of experts, such as peers with expertise in medical, statistical or research areas. This type of external committee may be appointed as an impartial panel to oversee the scientific and ethical integrity of a research study.[3] As such, an external committee can direct the progress of a research study, approve interim analyses and advise in decision-making processes about important matters such as whether to change the study protocol or stop the study. For example, the monitoring committee can direct interim analyses to confirm sample size requirements, can oversee safety analyses to investigate unexpected adverse events and can make decisions about the continuation of the study.

A monitoring committee may also have the responsibility of putting procedures in place to ensure the integrity of the database, the quality of the data entry, and other important aspects such as data security arrangements and documentation. All studies should have a management committee that is responsible for planning the data analyses and the publication of results prior to the data collection being completed or the study code being broken.

Team management

Managing a research team is no different from managing any other type of team. Most well balanced teams have a diversity of skills and personalities, and have systems in place to make group decisions and problem-solve on a regular and ongoing basis. It is important to create a culture of personal satisfaction by conducting a study in the best way possible so that the staff are proud to be involved. It is also important to create a purpose orientated working environment in which roles and responsibilities are clearly defined. This will help to foster an atmosphere in which people enjoy working together and being supportive of one another.

Some of the basic principles of effective team management are shown in Table 5.3. Good team management will ensure a more positive workplace atmosphere and will encourage greater personal commitment from the team members. This is an important component in the chain of activities that lead to the conduct of high quality research studies.

Table 5.3   Team management

- maintain a reliable level of trust and credibility
- encourage a commitment to quality data and research practices
- set realistic priorities
- ensure balance between interesting and mundane tasks for all team members
- encourage staff to take responsibility for tasks they enjoy most
- recognise that everyone in the team contributes to the final results
- hold regular meetings to foster good communication and co-operative problem solving skills
- ensure that team members have clearly defined roles and responsibilities
- have a clear management structure and methods for dealing with problems
- focus on personal achievements and professional development
- celebrate successes

Health science research

Remember that regular meetings and regular interactions within the study team not only facilitate the decision-making process but also foster a sense of teamwork and belonging. It is also important to foster good communications in order to create a positive flow of information between team members. These systems help to facilitate good science, which in turn contributes to the establishment of good research reputations.

Research skills

Research staff who are good team members usually turn out to be the people who are able to take responsibility for their own mistakes, which can happen at all levels of management and data collection, and are able to learn from them. In facilitating this process, it is important that all research staff are actively involved in the decision-making processes of the study so that they feel able to accept decisions that are taken to ensure the scientific integrity of the study. In this way, research staff can be acknowledged as professional workers who have the knowledge required for their work and who are committed to the best interests of the research project. The staff who are highly competent and professional, who find their job rewarding and who gain fulfilment from being part of a research team are most likely to collect research data to a high scientific standard. This will ensure that the study hypotheses can be tested in the best way possible.

It is essential that the study co-ordinator is familiar with all aspects of the study. It is also important that this person is pro-active and works to make life easier for the data collectors and study managers.[4] This will involve all aspects of facilitating subject recruitment and follow-up including identifying and solving day-to-day problems, tracking and organising the paperwork, keeping adequate stores of equipment and goods required, and making constant checks on data quality. This role can only be undertaken by a person who is both professional and competent, and who likes their job and enjoys helping other people.

Section 2—Randomisation methods

The objectives of this section are to understand:

- why randomisation is important;
- how to design a randomised study;
- how to select subjects randomly from a population;
- how to allocate subjects randomly to a study group;
- how to produce even numbers in the study groups; and
- how to deal with clusters in the randomisation process.

Randomisation

Randomisation is used in two situations in research; that is, in randomly selecting subjects to ensure that they are a representative sample of the general population or of a specific group of patients, or in randomly allocating subjects to different study groups in order to minimise the effects of confounding. Whatever the situation, it is important that the methods used to achieve randomisation are carefully chosen to ensure that any systematic bias is minimised. Randomisation is such an important aspect of clinical trials that some journals have a policy of declining to publish studies in which the allocation processes have not been properly randomised.[5]

The methods that can be used to randomly select subjects for inclusion in a study, to randomly allocate subjects to treatment groups and then conceal the allocation methods from the researchers who are responsible for collecting the data, are shown in Table 5.4.

Table 5.4 Random selection and random allocation	
Random selection	Random number table or computer generated sequence
Random allocation—unbalanced	
Simple randomisation	Random number table or computer generated sequence
Quasi-randomisation	Selection by age, date, number etc.
Random allocation—balanced	
Restricted randomisation	Allocation by sealed envelopes
Block randomisation	Randomisation in small blocks
Replacement randomisation	Sequences that exceed balance are rejected
Dynamic balanced randomisation	Allocation forced when groups unbalanced
Biased coin randomisation	Probability changed when groups unbalanced
Minimisation	Allocation by prognostic factors when groups unbalanced

Random selection

Random selection of subjects is the most effective method to reduce sampling error and therefore to ensure representativeness of the sample in order to maximise generalisability. In general, selection is from an ordered list in which each unit, such as the subjects, schools, towns, GP practices etc., has a unique identifying number. The unique numbers are then selected randomly from the list.

Glossary

Term	Meaning
Sampling frame	Target population from whom a sample is selected
Study strata	Subsets of sample divided according to a group e.g. age or gender
Imbalance	Failure to produce equal numbers in the study groups

If the number of units that are included in the sampling frame is less than 100, then a random number table, which can be found in most statistics books, may be the simplest method to use. It is important to decide a pattern for extracting numbers before beginning, for example the table can be read by row, by column or by block. Once the pattern has been decided, it has to be maintained until a sequence of sufficient length is obtained. To begin, a starting point in the table is chosen, and the random number sequence that is generated is used to select subjects by their serial numbers in the order that the numbers are selected. If a number is generated that has already been selected, it is discarded.

For randomly selecting subjects from a list of more than 100 people, it is more efficient to use a random number sequence that is generated using computer software. The procedure for doing this using Excel software is shown in Table 5.5. Other statistical software packages can also be used in a similar way. Once the sequence is obtained, the subjects are selected by beginning at the top of the randomised sequence and selecting subjects whose identification number matches the random number. Because any duplicates in the list have to be ignored, it is a good idea to generate a list that is longer than anticipated.

Table 5.5   Steps to generate a random number sequence using Excel
software

To generate then numbers
❏ Use Tools, Data analysis, Random number generator
❏ Number of variables = 1
❏ Number of random numbers = 100 (or however many are needed)
❏ Distribution = Uniform
❏ Parameters, Between = 1 to 4 if there are 4 groups to be allocated or 1 to 200 if there are 200 subjects in the list—this parameter indicates the highest number required
❏ Random seed = enter a different number each time, e.g. 123, 345, etc.
❏ New worksheet = a1:a100 to complement number needed
To round the numbers
❏ Highlight the column of numbers
❏ Use Format, Cells
❏ Number, Decimal places = 0

For example, to select six names at random from the list of names in Table 5.6, a random number sequence is first generated. Using Excel random number generator as shown in Table 5.5, the first random sequence that is generated is 2, 3, 19, 13, 3, 4, 3, 19, 8, ... The duplicate numbers in the sequence, which are 3, 3 and 19, are ignored. The resulting six randomly selected subjects are shown with an asterisk. When selecting randomly from a list, the order of the list is of no concern. It does not matter whether the list is ordered alphabetically, by date, or simply in the sequence in which subjects present.

No.	Name	No.	Name
Table 5.6 List of names and numbers			
1	Broderick J	11	Leslie T
2 *	Park J	12	Yoon H
3	McDonald D	13 *	Dixon D
4 *	Wenham D	14	Border A
5	Honnosay A	15	Johnson T
6	McKenna C	16	Black J
7	Thompson A	17	Fernando M
8 *	Muller S	18	McLelland J
9	Martin K	19 *	Brown N
10	King G	20	Mitchell J

Random allocation

Random allocation is the process of randomly allocating subjects to two or more study groups. This is the most effective method of removing the influence of both known and unknown confounders. Thus, clinical trials in which randomisation is used to allocate subjects to treatment groups are better able to answer questions about the efficacy or effectiveness of treatments. Although it is possible to compensate for the influence of known confounders and prognostic factors in the analyses, post-hoc methods conducted using multivariate data analyses are less efficient and cannot compensate for factors that are not known or have not been measured. The failure to use effective randomisation procedures can result in otherwise satisfactory studies being rejected for publication.[6]

When randomly allocating subjects to a study group, it is important to use a method that generates an unpredictable allocation sequence. It may also be important to produce balanced numbers in the study groups, especially when they are distributed between different study groups or centres. Once random allocation has been achieved, it is essential to have a protocol to conceal the random allocation methods from the research team so that they remain blinded to the potential study group of all subjects who are being recruited. Methods to achieve allocation concealment are presented in Chapter 2. The essential features of random allocation and concealment are shown in Table 5.7.

Table 5.7   Features of random allocation and concealment

- ensures that each subject has an equal chance of being allocated to each group
- ensures that differences between groups are due to treatment and not to differences in the distribution of prognostic factors or confounders
- are superior to systematic methods that allow the investigator to be 'unblinded'
- the allocation code is not available before the subject has been assessed as eligible and has consented to participate
- the research team responsible for subject recruitment is blinded to the methods of random allocation until recruitment is complete

---

Simple randomisation

Simple randomisation, which is also called *complete unbalanced* or *unrestricted randomisation*, is the gold standard in random allocation. The process is shown in Figure 5.1. The random sequence can be generated by tossing a coin but this is not recommended. A better method is to use a random number table or a random number sequence generated by computer software. For allocating a relatively small number of subjects to treatment groups, a random number table may be the simplest method to use.

Figure 5.1   Method of simple randomisation

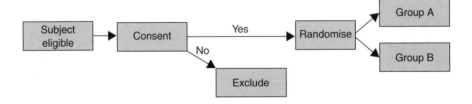

When using a random number table, the interpretation of the two digit numbers that are given by the table first needs to be decided. The choices are to use both digits as one number or, if numbers of 10 and over are not required, to use either the first digit, the second digit or both digits. For example, a sequence of

$$34 \ 15 \ 09$$

can be used as

34, 15, 9
3, 4, 1, 5, 0, 9
3, 1, 0
4, 5, 9

The pre-determined selection sequence can then be used to allocate subjects to the study groups. An example of how the numbers might be used is shown in Table 5.8. Similar sequences can be used for a larger number of groups.

The advantage of simple randomisation is that it balances prognostic factors perfectly between the study groups, provided that the sample size is large enough. A disadvantage is that it may result in uneven numbers in each group, especially if the sample size is small. Imbalance of subject numbers in different treatment groups is more of a problem in small studies in that the result may be difficult to interpret if the groups are very different in size. This problem is shown in Example 5.1.

However, imbalance is less of a problem in large studies in which the degree of imbalance will always be small in relation to the sample size. Remember that imbalance affects efficiency because a larger number of subjects will need to be recruited in order to maintain the same statistical power. Also, if imbalance is unpredictable between different study centres, then bias due to recruitment and measurement practices at each centre cannot be ruled out.

Table 5.8	Use of random numbers to allocate subjects to groups	
	Number	Group
Method 1	0–4	A
	5–9	B
Method 2	1, 3, 5, 7, 9	A
	2, 4, 6, 8, 0	B
Method 3	1–3	A
	4–6	B
	7–9	C
	0	Ignore

Example 5.1 Inadvertent unequal randomisation in a clinical trial Quinlan et al. Vitamin A and respiratory syncitial virus infection[7]	
Characteristic	Description
Aim	To determine whether oral vitamin A supplementation reduces symptoms in children with respiratory syncitial virus (RSV)
Type of study	Randomised controlled trial
Sample base	Children recruited from a hospital setting
Subjects	32 RSV infected patients age 2–58 months randomised to receive treatment or placebo 35 inpatient controls with no respiratory infection and 39 healthy outpatient controls
Treatment	21 children in RSV group received a single dose of oral vitamin A and 11 received placebo; allocation by randomisation
Outcome measurements	Serum vitamin A and retinol binding protein levels Clinical indicators of severity, e.g. days of hospitalisation, oxygen use, intensive care, intubation and daily severity scores
Statistics	T-tests, Fisher's exact test, ANOVA and non-parametric tests
Conclusion	• no benefit of vitamin A supplementation in children hospitalised for RSV • children hospitalised with RSV had lower serum vitamin A and retinol binding protein levels than outpatient control subjects
Strengths	• efficacy of a simple intervention to reduce severity of RSV not known • two external control groups enrolled
Limitations	• description of randomisation method as being carried out in relatively large blocks and resultant imbalance in group numbers suggests that randomisation was not achieved • only one-third of sample base enrolled therefore generalisability limited • blood unable to be obtained for 10 of the 32 children in the randomised controlled trial therefore serum outcome data could not be evaluated

Cont'd

Example 5.1 Cont'd   Inadvertent unequal randomisation in a clinical trial

Characteristic	Description
	• small numbers in randomised trial resulted in a lack of statistical power to test for clinically important differences in most outcome measurements between groups

Quasi-randomisation

Quasi-randomisation, or systematic assignment, involves allocating subjects to a study group using available numbers such as their birth date, medical record number or the day of the week. This method is sometimes used for convenience but does not guarantee the balance of confounders between groups. In fact, these types of methods are likely to increase bias because the group is not determined entirely by chance and the group allocation is extremely difficult to conceal. Knowledge of group allocation when a patient is being considered for entry into a study may influence the decision on the part of the research staff whether to recruit that patient to a particular study group. Any practices that result in the differential recruitment or allocation of subjects are likely to lead to treatment groups in which important confounders are not balanced.[8]

Restricted randomisation

In small studies, imbalance can be overcome by restricted randomisation. For this, opaque envelopes with equal numbers of cases and controls are prepared, manually shuffled, and then given a sequential number. The envelopes are then opened in sequence as each subject is recruited. For stratification (for example by gender or by age group), two colours of envelopes or two types of identifying labels can be used.

This type of randomisation is not a preferred method because there is a large potential for non-concealment. For example, envelopes may be transparent or may be opened prior to the subject giving consent to be entered into the study. In addition, the predictability of the group allocation may increase towards the end of the study. Say, for example, that four subjects remain to be recruited and that group A has four more subjects already allocated than group B. In situations such as this, it is clear that the remaining recruits will be allocated to group B to produce equal study groups. If the observers are not blinded to study group, there is a potential for selection bias to be introduced if some subjects are recruited because of a perception that they are more 'suitable' for certain groups.

Block randomisation

The basis of block randomisation is that subjects are randomised within small groups, that is in blocks, of say, three, four or six subjects. This method is most useful for random allocation in large studies or multi-centre trials in which an equal number of subjects need to be allocated to each group in each centre. The basis of the random allocation is to generate all possible combinations of the group allocation sequence for the block size that is selected.

For example, for a block size of four subjects who are being allocated to one of two treatments, there are six sequences in which we could allocate subjects to either treatment A or treatment B, that is AABB, ABAB, ABBA, BABA, BAAB and BBAA. To undertake block randomisation, these sequences are numbered from one to six and selected randomly, as discussed in the random selection section above, to determine the order in which they are used for allocation. Each consecutive sequence determines the group allocation of the next four subjects.

An example of block randomisation using a block size of three units to randomly allocate subjects to three different groups A, B and C at one time is shown in Table 5.9. The process involves first numbering all possible sequences in which the allocation of subjects to groups could occur, then using unbalanced randomisation to select the order of the sequences that will be used. This method has the advantage that it ensures that group numbers are balanced after any number of allocations and it can be used for both simple and stratified randomisation.

Table 5.9   Randomisation by blocks

For a block size of 3, the following combinations of 3 groups are possible:
1. ABC
2. ACB
3. BAC
4. BCA
5. CAB
6. CBA

If the order of numbers selected randomly is 6, 2, 3, 6, 1 etc. then the order of allocation of subjects to groups is CBA ACB BAC CBA ABC etc.

A disadvantage with block randomisation is that the block size may become obvious to the observers so that concealment is lost for a significant proportion of subjects. If a study is relatively small, then a block size of less than six can be discerned from the pattern of past allocations. A method to prevent this is to occasionally change the block size over the course of the study as an added measure to safeguard concealment. Thus, a block size of three may be used for the first three subjects, five for the next five subjects, four for the next four subjects etc.

Although the practice of block randomisation is effective for small block sizes, it can become complex when larger block sizes that have many possible combinations are used. For example, if a block size of ten is chosen for randomising subjects to only two treatment groups, there are 252 possible sequences. However, for studies with only two treatment groups, the allocation process is simpler. For example, if the block size is six, then simple randomisation can be used to allocate three subjects to group A and the remainder are placed in group B. Thus, if three random numbers four, three, one are selected from a table, the allocation of the first six subjects would be ABAABB. This process is then repeated for each successive block. The study presented in Example 2.4[9] in Chapter 2 used block randomisation in a pragmatic clinical trial and resulted in the numbers of subjects in study groups shown in Figure 5.2.

Figure 5.2   Outcome of recruitment and randomisation strategy

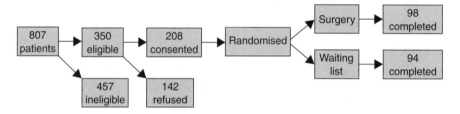

Replacement randomisation

In replacement randomisation, a maximum imbalance between groups is pre-specified and sequences that exceed the imbalance are rejected.[10] Using this method, new sequences are continually generated using simple randomisation until a random sequence that meets the specification is met. Table 5.10 shows a situation in which the first set of random numbers generated produced nine subjects in group A and six in group B, and the second set produced five in group A and ten in group B. Both produced an imbalance that was greater than the pre-specified criteria of two. The third sequence, which produced seven subjects in group A and eight in group B, was the first acceptable sequence.

Table 5.10	Three sequential treatment assignments using replacement randomisation														
Subject No:	1	2	3	4	5	6	7	8	9	10	11	12	13	14	15
1st set	A	A	A	B	B	B	A	B	A	A	A	B	A	B	A
2nd set	A	A	B	A	B	B	B	A	B	B	A	B	B	B	B
3rd set	A	A	B	B	A	A	B	A	B	A	B	A	B	B	B

The disadvantage of all balanced random allocations is that they are easily unblinded in the final stages of trial. For example in the 3rd set in Table 5.10, which was the first acceptable set, the first twelve allocations produced seven subjects in group A and five in group B. From this, it could easily be guessed that at least two of the remaining three would in all likelihood be allocated to group B. This method is only suitable for small studies with few treatment groups because the number of replacements that are required become larger as the group size increases and the sample size decreases.

However, the advantages of replacement randomisation are that it guarantees an upper boundary on imbalance, the method is easy to implement and the assignments remain more unpredictable than for block randomisation. In addition, this method can be used in stratified trials although the total imbalance limit across the study may need to be considered.

Biased coin randomisation

Biased coin randomisation, which is also called *adaptive* randomisation, is a randomisation method in which the probability of assigning subjects to each group is altered at points when the groups become unbalanced. At the point when groups become unbalanced, the probability of a subject being assigned to the group with the least number of subjects is increased. An example of biased coin randomisation is shown in Figure 5.3. In this example, 4:6 ratio of allocating subjects to groups B and A is used when group A is larger than group B, but an equal probability when the group sizes are equal.

Figure 5.3 Biased coin randomisation

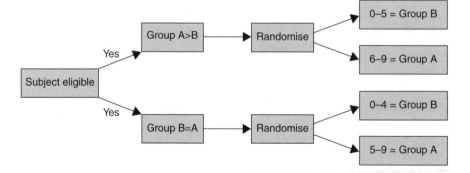

Probability theory shows that changing to a probability of 3/4 maintains the best control over imbalance. Because this may be predictable once an imbalance exists, changing to a probability of 2/3 for small studies or 3/5 for larger studies is preferred.[11] For example, suppose that numbers 0–4 are used to allocate subjects to group A and 5–9 are used for group B but only at points when the size of groups A and B are equal. At all other times, the numbers 0–5 (i.e. $P=3/5$) will be used to assign subjects to the group with the smaller number of subjects and the numbers 6–9 (i.e. $P=2/5$) will be used to assign subjects to the group with the larger number of subjects. Table 5.11 shows an example in which biased coin randomisation is used to balance two groups in a study.

Table 5.11	Allocation sequence using biased coin randomisation with $P=3/5$															
Random number	1	5*	4	5*	8	7	3	2*	4	1*	6	8	3	8	5	0*
Group	A	B	A	B	B	B	A	A	A	D	D	B	A	B	A	A
A/B	1/0	1/1	2/1	2/2	2/3	2/4	3/4	4/4	5/4	5/5	5/6	5/7	6/7	6/8	7/8	8/8

* when groups are equal 0–4=A and 5–9=B, otherwise 0–5=smaller group and 6–9=larger group

This method can also be used when the imbalance exceeds a pre-specified limit, say when the imbalance between groups exceeds three. For studies with more than two groups, the method becomes complex and block randomisation is much simpler to administer.

Glossary

Term	Meaning
Selection bias	Distortion in the results caused by non-random methods to select the subjects
Allocation bias	Distortion in the results caused by the processes of allocating subjects to a case or control group

Minimisation

Minimisation is a method of randomisation that ensures that any prognostic factors are balanced between study groups. This method is especially useful for balancing subject numbers over two or more levels of important characteristics. This can be a critical issue in small clinical trials in which a large difference in important confounders between groups can occur purely by chance.[12] If this happens, it becomes difficult to decide whether differences between the groups can be ascribed to the treatment in question or are largely due to the imbalance in prognostic factors. Imbalance also has the potential to reduce the statistical power of large clinical trials that are designed to measure small differences between study groups.

To use minimisation, a tally of the number of subjects in each of the subgroups has to be continually updated. Before the study begins, the important prognostic characteristics are listed and then, during enrolment, the running total of the numbers is used to decide group allocation of the next subject.[13] From Table 5.12, the sum of the top rows for each factor in the table is calculated. Thus, the sums are as follows:

$$Group\ A = 20 + 12 + 20 = 52$$

$$Group\ B = 19 + 8 + 16 = 43$$

In this situation, the next patient would be allocated to group B, which has the lowest total. At points when the two totals are equal, simple randomisation would be used.

Table 5.12	Group assignment for 55 subjects using minimisation				
		Group A	Group B	Subgroup total	Group total
Age	<40 yrs	20	19	39	55
	≥40 yrs	8	8	16	
Gender	Male	12	8	20	55
	Female	22	13	35	
Smoking	No	20	16	36	55
	Yes	8	11	19	

Minimisation ensures similarity between the groups. At the point of entry into the study, each subject is assigned to the group with the lowest frequency of their characteristics. For example, if smoking predicts outcome then a smoker would be assigned to the group that has the lowest proportion of smokers already enrolled. However, as the number of strata increase, the complexity of this method increases. For example, for three strata with two levels in each as shown in Table 5.12, a total of six groups have to be balanced. Alternatively, the odds for entry into each group can be changed as described in the biased coin method so that an element of chance always remains. At points of balance, simple randomisation is again used. A disadvantage with the use of minimisation in small studies is that specific strata may not have a balance of treatment groups and thus any effects of confounders will be poorly controlled.

Dynamic balanced randomisation

A method of randomisation that can be useful in unblinded studies is dynamic balanced randomisation.[14] This method is a variation of replacement randomisation in that unbalanced randomisation is used until a critical, pre-specified imbalance is reached after which subjects are assigned to the group with the smallest enrolment number in order to redress the imbalance. The method of this type of randomisation is shown in Figure 5.4. The advantage of this method is that it is simple to use in studies in which randomisation by several strata is required and for which other methods become complex to administer. Dynamic balanced randomisation balances the numbers of treatment allocations within groups whilst retaining an element of randomisation. The disadvantage is that concealment is easily unblinded once an imbalance is reached.

Figure 5.4   Dynamic balanced randomisation

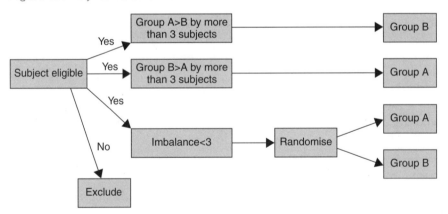

In some situations, this method has advantages over randomised block designs, which can become predictable if the researchers who are recruiting subjects have deduced the block size, or minimisation, which can be poor in controlling for confounding in specific groups of subjects. Dynamic balanced randomisation reduces imbalance, results in a smaller risk of selection bias than randomised block designs and may offer greater protection against unbalanced group numbers than is achieved with minimisation.

Unequal randomisation

Clinical trials with an equal number of subjects in each group are most efficient in terms of the total number of subjects who need to be enrolled to answer the study questions. However, if a new treatment is being compared to a currently used treatment, then a larger number of subjects are sometimes randomised to the new treatment group. This type of unequal randomisation is often used when there is a need to gain experience with the new treatment including collecting information about possible advantages and disadvantages with its use. If the ratio of new treatment to standard treatment subjects is 2:1 or 3:2, the small loss of statistical power may be balanced by the value of the information gained. However, a randomisation ratio greater than 3:1 becomes quite inefficient.[15]

Methods for randomising to groups of unequal size require adaptation of the methods discussed above. For example, if simple randomisation is used then numbers 1–6 may be used to assign subjects to the new treatment group, 7–9 to the standard treatment group and 0 ignored. For randomising in a 2:1 ratio using block randomisation, subjects can be randomised to three groups as shown above where A and B are the new treatment group and C is the standard treatment group. Similar adaptations of other methods can also be made.

Randomisation in clusters

In epidemiological studies, subjects are often selected or allocated to study groups in clusters. For example, when selecting children from a population in order to measure the prevalence of a disease, the schools often form the sampling frame and are selected as units, rather than randomising the individual children within them.

For many types of community interventions, it is simply not feasible to randomise individual participants to different study groups. In studies to test the effectiveness of an intervention in communities, it is common to randomise individual communities to receive the active or control treatment. For example, in a study of the impact of fly control on childhood diarrhoea in Pakistan, six study villages were randomly assigned to two study groups.[16] The problem with this type of randomisation is that it does not control for possible differences between the communities. In the study in the example, this was partly overcome with the use of a cross-over study design, in that three of the villages were sprayed in the first year and the remaining three in the second year. Despite the limitations in the study design, cluster randomisation is often the only practical method with which to gain information of whether community interventions have potential benefits to health.

Health science research

Cluster randomisation is also sometimes used to randomise clinical practices to arms of an intervention. In this situation, all subjects within a practice will be in the same treatment arm. This procedure is effective in maintaining subject blinding by decreasing the likelihood that patients in different groups will interact with one another. However, in this type of study, the analyses have to take account of both the variation between subjects and the variation between practices. One of the major limitations in cluster designs is that this approach leads to a loss of efficiency and statistical power.

Cluster designs are not such a problem in studies in which the number of practices is large and the number of subjects per practice is quite small. However, in studies in which there are only a small number of practices or in which the number of subjects per practice is large, any analyses that ignore the clusters will tend to under-estimate the standard error of the treatment effect.[17] A simple method to take account of the clusters is to calculate a summary measure of the outcome variable for each practice and to use that in the analyses. In this type of analysis, the effective sample size is the number of practices and not the number of subjects. A disadvantage with this approach is that the standard error will be over-inflated and a type II error may occur if the number of units is small.

Section 3—Data management

The objectives of this section are to understand:
- how to manage the data collected during a research study;
- how to minimise errors in the results; and
- the importance of security and subject confidentiality.

Steps in data management

All studies, no matter what type of study design is used, require a high standard of accuracy in storing the research data. To achieve this, a series of logical steps in data management must be followed before data analyses begin. A checklist for this process is shown in Table 5.13. In order to progress in this way, it is important to develop a timeline and leave enough time to complete each step diligently. There is always a temptation to jump in and analyse new data files as soon as they become available. However, the results from this type of approach may be spurious if the data have not been treated carefully, and it is unethical to mislead others by reporting results that turn out to be a mistake at a later date.

Table 5.13   Checklist for managing data
❑ Code data appropriately
❑ Enter data into a database
❑ Conduct range and visual checks
❑ Make all corrections that are needed
❑ Check for duplicate records in key fields

Cont'd

Table 5.13 Cont'd   Checklist for managing data

❑ Merge data from different instruments if they have been used
❑ Archive a copy of the database in a safe, fireproof place
❑ Limit access to sensitive data

Database design

For statistical analysis, the data will need to be entered into a database. Although database design is time-consuming, it is important that this task is the responsibility of someone who has established database skills because small errors and inconsistencies at the planning stage can lead to insurmountable difficulties during the data analyses.

It is much better to enter data into a well-designed database than to enter it directly into an electronic spreadsheet. An advantage of using a database is that it forces the person who is responsible for managing the data to address many of the essential data management issues before the data are entered. This not only facilitates the integrity of the data but is also an efficient process because it simplifies the data analyses at a later stage. The issues that need to be considered when designing a database are shown in Table 5.14. The type, physical length (size) and categorisation of each variable are essential features that need to be defined. By defining the data correctly and using cross-checks to ensure that values outside permitted ranges are not admissible, the quality of the data will be optimised.

Table 5.14   Issues to consider when designing a database
• data type, e.g. numeric, alphabetic, binary, date, etc.
• data size or maximum allowable length
• permitted categories, or permitted range of values
• definitions of pre-determined study groups
• coding to identify sub-categories of explanatory variables
• validation of permitted values
• codes to identify missing data

Remember that, if an item needs to be recoded in order to categorise subjects by an accepted definition, the original data should be entered into the database rather than the recoded version. This will maintain flexibility to adjust for changes in the definition at a later stage. For example, an epidemiological definition that was widely used for many years to define the presence of airway abnormalities associated with asthma was a 20 per cent fall in lung function after administering 7.8 μmol of histamine. However, following large-scale validation studies, this was later changed to a 20 per cent fall at 3.9 μmol histamine. By entering the original data, the definition could be changed by reclassifying subjects at a later date so that a valid comparison could be made between the results from the historical and contemporary studies. This would not have been possible if a binary response of a positive or negative result was the only data that had been stored in the database.

Data entry

Data entry is a simple task if self-coding questionnaires have been used but, if not, decisions about whether to enter items as alphabetic or numeric information will need to be made. Data must be thoroughly checked and corrected before being entered into the database, and any further errors that require correction should be dealt with as soon as possible. If data entry is undertaken soon after the subject is studied, any ambiguous or missing information can be replaced by contacting the subject to verify the data. Also, if data collection is ongoing, information of recurring errors can lead to more accurate data collection techniques being developed for use in the remainder of the study.

Data entered into a computer database must always be verified, that is checked by a second operator, to ensure they are correct. Commercial companies often 'double enter' the data for this purpose. If this procedure is not adopted, then a random one in five or one in ten sample of the data should be re-entered by an operator who is blinded to the initial data entry values. The two databases can then be cross-checked to identify the rate of occurrence of any inconsistencies in data entry. All errors that are detected in a research database, together with details about their corrections, should be recorded in the data management manual.

If data are commercially entered they will need to be exported (sent back to you) in a suitable format. The most versatile format is 'comma delimited', i.e. the items are separated in the electronic file by commas, because this can be easily read into most programs. An alternative format is 'tab delimited' and can be read by most programs but because this format requires extra storage space, it is only practical if the records for each subject are quite short. If the records are long, it may be better to use 'field format' with each data item appearing in a set column and without any gaps left between fields. In this case, the field positions need to be very carefully specified when importing the data into the database.

Alphabetic strings

Numeric coding usually simplifies data analysis because statistical packages and spreadsheets are primarily designed to handle this type of information. Although many packages can handle alphabetic strings, the strings need to be kept short and have to be case, length and spelling consistent. Some statistical packages are able to group subjects using alphabetic strings, but others are not so that the information has to be recoded eventually. Computer packages usually allow most types of data to be recoded if necessary, although the process can be tedious. In general, it is more time and cost effective for both data management and data analysis to code replies numerically at the time of data collection using efficient data recording forms (see Chapter 3). This maintains the efficiency of the study by minimising the amount of missing data and optimises repeatability and validity by minimising the number of errors and inconsistencies.

Missing values

For efficient data analyses, missing values should be given a non-numerical missing code so that they cannot be inadvertently incorporated into analyses. Missing values that are coded as '.' (i.e. a full stop) are preferable because they are consistently treated as missing values in all analyses. On the other hand, missing values that are coded as numeric values such as 0, 9 or 99 can be inadvertently incorporated into analyses. It is also important to decide if 'don't know' replies will be coded as negative responses or treated as missing values.

Database management

After the data are entered into the database, they need to be examined carefully using range checks to identify any outliers in the data. Other techniques such as sorting the data or conducting visual checks of data lists can be used to ensure any obvious inadvertent errors and illogical values have not occurred. This needs to be undertaken for all data sets, but especially when a commercial company or other data entry personnel who have no knowledge or insight into the meaning of the data values, have entered the data. In addition, if indirect methods of data entry are used, the accuracy of all fields in the database should be cross-checked to ensure that all transfers and recodes or recalculations are correct. Value labels and variable labels need to be coded into the database at this stage to ensure that all statistical output is self-documented.

If more than one instrument has been used to collect data, then several records may have to be matched together. To do this, it is important to match on at least two unique fields such as name and identification number. Matching by a single field alone is not enough to ensure that errors in collation do not occur. Before matching begins, be sure to check for duplicates in all of the key fields being used.

Connectivity software

Connectivity software is a computer facility that allows statistical and spreadsheet packages to 'look into' the database and read the data. For research purposes, a relational database is the most appropriate method for storing data. If connectivity software is available, an added advantage of using a relational database is that the data can be analysed directly without being exported to another file and then imported into specialist statistical software.

The use of connectivity software prevents the need for multiple versions of the data being stored as separate files and, as such, ensures optimal data integrity at all stages in the data collection, data management and data analyses processes. To facilitate summarising or analysing the data, the database can be accessed in read-only mode to protect its integrity. Moreover, data analyses can be very readily updated following any corrections or additions to the data set. This approach also circumvents the processes of exporting, importing and documenting various versions of data sets at several points during the data analyses. The investment made in setting up a relational database and becoming competent in methods of using connectivity software are more than offset by an increased confidence in the data analyses and in the results.

Security and subject confidentiality

The security of the database will need to be addressed in terms of access by other users, subject confidentiality and back-up in case of loss. In order that the data in the database cannot be altered inadvertently, the write privileges of the researchers who need to access the database can be restricted.

Only one master database for each data set should be maintained, and this should be the entire data set in which all errors are corrected, as they become obvious. An archived copy of the final, corrected database can then be used reliably at a later date, for example for a follow-up study. At all times, a back-up (duplicate) copy of the master database must be kept in safe storage in case of fire, theft or computer failure. In institutions where a computer network is in place, this process is often the responsibility of the computer department.

Exporting data for data analyses

When connectivity software is not available, abbreviated working files or spreadsheets can be created for undertaking essential clerical tasks and data analyses. In such situations, corrections should always be made on the main file so that a single, high quality master database is maintained at all times.

Working files are often abbreviated files that do not have identifying or contact information of the study subjects or information that is not being used in specific analyses. In their shortened forms, working files save computing time during data analyses. To maintain subject confidentiality and ethics agreements, fields that identify the subject can be omitted from work files and made invisible to people who have access to the database.

6

ANALYSING THE DATA

Section 1—Planning analyses
Section 2—Statistical methods

Section 1—Planning analyses

The objectives of this section are to understand how to:
- plan the data analysis stage of a research study;
- deal with missing data and errors;
- categorise variables for statistical analysis; and
- document the process of data management and analysis.

Sequence for data analysis

Analysing the data and interpreting the results is one of the most exciting stages in a research study because this provides the answers to the study questions. However, this stage is one of the crucial stages in the quest for truth so it is important that the process is undertaken in a careful and considered way.

There have been many examples of results being published and the conclusions then being reversed following a later re-analysis of the data.[1] To avoid this, it is important that data are treated carefully and analysed slowly by people who are familiar with their content and their nature. Data analyses also need to be planned and undertaken in a logical and considered sequence to avoid errors or misinterpretation.

It is especially important that all steps in data analyses are documented so that anyone can see how the results were obtained. This is easily achieved by maintaining a log book in which programs that are run to obtain results are recorded together with the results of the data analyses and the date that they were generated, and information of the location and documentation of the files. With this approach, the results of analyses can be easily back-tracked and cross-checked if any anomalies become apparent.

When analysing data, it is always prudent to tread a conservative path and to maintain scientific correctness when considering procedures such as omitting records, recoding outliers or re-grouping data, and when choosing the types of analysis that will be used. Keep in mind that it is misleading, and perhaps unethical, to use numbers in a way that produces statistically significant but clinically spurious results. Conversely, it is extremely satisfying and professional to conclude a study in the knowledge that the data have been correctly analysed and reported. The sequential procedures for data analysis are discussed below and are shown as a checklist in Table 6.1.

Table 6.1   Checklist for analysing data
Univariate analyses
❑ Conduct distribution and frequency checks of variables
❑ Deal with missing values and outliers
❑ Recode groups and transform continuous variables if necessary
❑ Re-run distribution and frequency checks
❑ Document variable profiles in study handbook
Bivariate and multivariate analyses
❑ Categorise information into outcome, intervening or explanatory variables
❑ Conduct bivariate analyses to test for significant associations
❑ Check pair-wise plots for non-linearity and for outliers
❑ Limit analyses to those needed to test prior hypotheses
❑ Undertake multivariate analyses

Beginning the analyses

In general, any data analyses should progress through the logical steps of first conducting univariate analyses before progressing to the bivariate and then the multivariate analyses. By conducting univariate analyses before beginning any bivariate analyses, frequency distributions and content of each variable can be carefully inspected. This allows the data analyst to become familiar with the nature of data and gain insight into the range of values, possible miscoded or missing data, and any skewness in each variable. Without doing this, anomalies in the results of analyses may not always be obvious. When data are not normally distributed, transformations or the use of non-parametric statistics will be required. Once the data are corrected or transformed, information on their ranges and summary statistics should be stored in the data log book for future reference.

Missing data

Missing data must be treated very carefully. Missed data that occur in a random pattern reduce statistical power but rarely affect the results. However, missing data that occur in a non-random pattern may affect generalisability. For example, if people in high income brackets consistently omit to reply to a question about their salary range, then the results that are categorised by this variable can only be generalised to people in lower income brackets. The extent to which this type of bias is unacceptable can be assessed by examining the differences in outcome values or in the proportion of subjects with a disease in the groups with and without missing data.

Data with missing values should always be included in statistics such as prevalence rates but usually have to be excluded from bivariate or multivariate analyses. For continuous data, missing values can sometimes be substituted with a median or mean value. Using the mean for the total sample is a conservative substitution that leads to a loss of variance in the data. However, use of the subgroup mean or median is a less conservative approach.

Outliers

Outliers may be incorrect values or may be anomalies. Because these values have a larger influence on summary statistics than each of the valid data points, they have the potential to lead to type I or type II errors especially when the sample size is small. If outliers are included in the analyses, it is possible that the results may not generalise to an average population because the summary statistics are over- or under-estimated. To remedy this, the outlying value can be deleted or replaced. If the value is replaced, it is probably better to recode it to a value closer to the mean so that it is not unduly influential.

Categorising variables

Before beginning any bivariate or multivariate analyses, the variables need to be categorised into the types shown in Table 6.2. This will help to avoid distortion or lack of precision in summary estimates that occur when variables are not considered appropriately. The appropriate methods for classifying variables and for including confounders and effect-modifiers in multivariate models are outlined in Chapter 3.

Table 6.2 Categorisation of variables for data analysis		
Variable	Alternative names	Axis for plots
Outcome variables	Dependent variables (DVs)	y-axis
Intervening variables	Secondary or alternative outcome variables	y-axis
Explanatory variables	Independent variables (IVs) Risk factors Exposure variables Predictors	x-axis

Documentation

Every stage in the process of collecting data, coding responses, and making decisions about data management must be documented clearly in a data management file. In addition to keeping information about file structures, file locations, coding protocols and treatment of missing values and outliers, print-outs of all analyses should be stored together with the data transformations that were used for each one. All print-outs should be labelled with a date and information of the file location. Science is a quest for truth, and it is important that fellow researchers can access a database and obtain identical results from repeat analyses in order to validate the findings or further explore the data.

Limiting the number of analyses

If the data are being accrued gradually, it is important to avoid bias that can be caused by undertaking sequential interim analyses. It is usual, and prudent, to wait until the data set is complete and has been edited and corrected before statistical analyses begin. The processes for reducing bias that occurs as a result of conducting interim analyses are discussed in Chapter 4.

Careful thought should also be given to using data for purposes for which it was not collected. This practice is often called 'data dredging' or 'fishing expeditions'. Analyses that test all possible relationships between all variables are much more likely to produce spurious information than analyses that test relationships that have a sound scientific background. Cross-sectional and case-control studies lend themselves most to these practices. To avoid random significant findings (type I errors), it is best to limit the analyses to those that provide information about the frequency distribution of the variables and that only test hypotheses that were formed prior to data analysis.

On the other hand, new ideas emerge over time and the use of existing data sets to explore new ideas can conserve resources and maximise efficiency. If the study design is appropriate, existing data can be used to explore possible relations between potential risk factors and outcomes, or to generate new hypotheses. The need to reduce the possibility of type I errors has to be balanced with the possibility of type II errors. The failure to detect an association if one exists, which may occur if the analysis is not conducted, can be considered to be a type II error.[2] Also, the reality is that adjustments for multiple comparisons in the form of reducing the critical P value to <0.01 or <0.001 do not allow for a valid comparison of the results from different studies.[3] If the data are of high quality, then the validity of results that were not anticipated at the beginning of the study will not be affected and the quality of the data does not change if another hypothesis is tested.[4]

When undertaking data analyses, it is clearly important to only test a hypothesis that has biological plausibility, whether it be a prior hypothesis or a new hypothesis that has arisen since the study began. This approach will conserve resources and stimulate research ideas whilst minimising the potential to provide misleading information.

Section 2—Statistical methods

The objectives of this section are to understand how to:
- use a logical pathway for conducting statistical analyses;
- decide which statistical tests to use;
- describe the accuracy of the estimates; and
- judge whether to adjust for baseline characteristics.

Statistical analyses

Conducting the statistical analyses can be one of the most exciting parts of a study. Once all of the error corrections to the data have been made, it is vital that the correct statistical analyses are used so that the results can be interpreted accurately and correctly. There are many excellent statistical books that explain how to conduct, understand and interpret the multitude of statistical tests that are available. This section is intended as a guide to proceeding logically through the data analyses stage of a study by handling the data correctly and by selecting the correct statistical test. When critically appraising a published study, the statistics pathways can also be used as a guide to deciding whether the correct statistics have been used.

In designing research studies, we often plan to select a sample of subjects and use their data as a 'best estimate' of the population from which they were sampled. Thus, we use statistical analyses to produce summary information for a sample of subjects. In practice though, statistics such as the mean value or prevalence rate that we obtain from our sample are usually slightly different from those of the population from which the subjects were drawn. This is known as 'sampling variability'. In this chapter, we describe the statistics that can be used to describe the characteristics of study samples and to make inferences about the population in general.

Univariate methods

The first step in data analysis is to examine the frequencies of the categorical variables and the distributions of the continuous variables. This process will lead to an inherent understanding of the nature of the data that has been collected and to selecting the correct statistics that must be used for the analyses.

Categorical data analyses

For categorical data, histograms and frequency counts will show whether any groups with small numbers need combining with other categories. These counts will also indicate whether chi-square statistics, non-parametric tests or exact statistics need to be used in analyses and, if chi-square is being used, whether Pearson's chi-square, a continuity-correction chi-square or Fisher's exact test is the appropriate method (Chapter 7). A pathway for deciding which chi-square test to use for categorical data is shown in Figure 6.1.

Figure 6.1 Pathway for analysis of categorical data

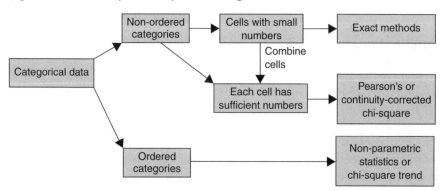

Categories with small numbers

Because categories with small numbers can have surprisingly large effects on statistical results, it is often prudent to merge some categories together if it makes sense to do so. This can be undertaken by inspecting the distribution of each variable to decide which cells need to be combined or where new boundaries for grouping variables are most sensibly created. To avoid post-hoc analyses, this procedure should be undertaken before any bivariate or multivariate analyses are performed.

The categories that are used in the data analyses must be meaningful and must preferably be in concordance with any prior evidence of effect. For example, if an effect has been shown to be different between subjects above and below the age of 35 years, then it is best not to divide the subjects into groups of <30 years, 30–39 years and ≥40 years of age. If the data are particularly sparse, the optimum number of categories will be two or three and it is unlikely that anything will be gained by maintaining a larger number. In multivariate analyses, an average of at least ten subjects in each cell in a contingency tabulation of the data is required. Table 6.3 shows how reducing each variable to a small number of categories helps to maintain statistical power.

Table 6.3 Increase in sample size required for multivariate analyses as the number of categories for each variable increases			
	Number of categories		
Disease outcome	2	2	3
Exposure variable	2	2	3
Confounder I	2	3	4
Confounder II	2	3	4
Number of cells in contingency table	16	36	144
Minimum sample size required	160	360	1440

Continuous data

When variables are continuous in nature, it is important to know whether they are normally distributed or whether the distribution is skewed. If the distribution does not approximate normality, then methods to transform the data need to be explored or non-parametric statistics will need to be used. In practice, it is preferable to use parametric statistics whenever possible because they provide greater statistical power than non-parametric statistics for the same sample size. A pathway for analysing continuous data is shown in Figure 6.2.

Figure 6.2 Pathway for analysis of continuous data

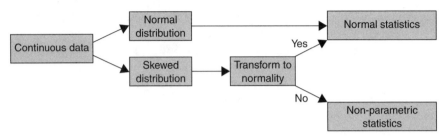

Much information about the distribution of continuous variables can be gained from simply calculating summary statistics such as the mean, standard deviation, median and range for each variable.[5] The data will be close to normally distributed if the mean is close to the centre of the range, that is the median value. It is also useful to inspect a frequency histogram of the data to assess whether the distribution is truly skewed or whether a few outliers are responsible for the mean and the median being unequal. Figures 6.3 and 6.4 show how the mean and median values are very close to one another for a normal distribution but become increasingly different if the distribution is skewed.

Figure 6.3 A normal distribution

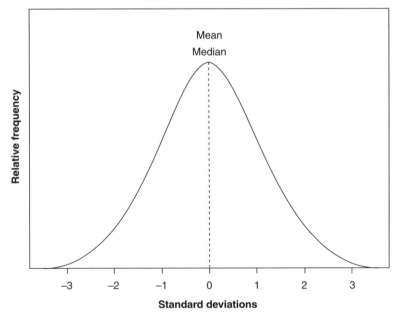

A normal distribution showing that the mean and median are identical.

Figure 6.4   A skewed data distribution

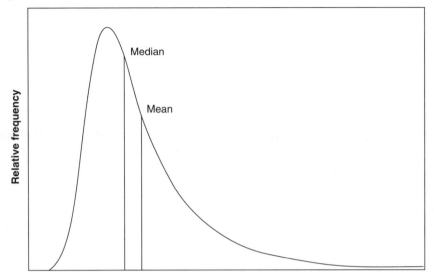

A skewed data distribution showing how the mean is an over-estimate of the median value, and is therefore not an accurate description of the centre of the distribution.

Glossary

Term	Interpretation	Meaning
Mean	Average value	Measure of the central tendency of the data
Median	'Centre' of data	Point at which half of the measurements lie below and half lie above this value
Standard deviation	Measure of spread	95% of the measurements lie within two standard deviations above and below the mean
Range	Measure of spread	Lowest to highest value
Standard error	Measure of precision	The interval of two standard errors above and below the mean indicates the range in which we can be 95% certain that the 'true' mean lies
95% confidence interval	Measure of precision	Interval around a summary statistic in which we are 95% certain that the 'true' estimate lies

Health science research

Because normal statistics do not describe skewed data with any accuracy, data that are not normally distributed have to be transformed to normality or non-parametric statistics need to be used. If the mean and median values are not known, as is often the case when judging published results, a useful trick to judge whether normal statistics are reliable for describing the data is to calculate the 95 per cent range as follows:

95% range = Mean − 2 SDs to Mean + 2 SDs

These two values should represent the range in which 95 per cent of the data points would lie if the measurement were normally distributed. If either of these two values is an important distance outside the true range of the measurements, then the distribution must be skewed. This problem can be seen in Example 6.1.

Example 6.1   Reporting of baseline characteristics[b]

% predicted normal value	Nebulizer group	Inhaler group	P
For FEV1	37.5 ± 16.6	36.1 ± 15.2	0.80
For FVC	55.4 ± 18.8	54.2 ± 18.4	0.86

The baseline characteristics of the lung function of the groups in the study shown in Example 2.3 in Chapter 2 were reported as the mean and 1 standard deviation as shown above. If the data were described well by these statistics, the 95% range of the FEV1 in the nebulizer group can be calculated as follows:

95% range = 37.5 ± (2 × 16.6)
= 4.3–70.7%

No subject could have an FEV1 as low as 4.3% of predicted. What is more likely is that there were a few subjects with very low values so that the data were skewed with a tail to the left and the mean underestimated the median value. In this case, the median and inter-quartile or absolute range would have been more accurate statistics with which to describe these data.

In addition, it was not necessary to undertake statistical tests and compute P values because the study hypothesis was not that the two groups would have different values. In fact, the P value will be inaccurate because a t-test has been used when the data are not normally distributed. A simple visual inspection of the data is sufficient to show that the two groups do not have a clinically important difference in terms of baseline lung function.

When reviewing journal articles in which only the standard error is given, the standard deviation can be simply derived using the formula:

$$SD = SE \times \sqrt{n}$$

If normal statistics have been used when the data are skewed, then the mean value will be inaccurate and the conclusions drawn from the results of the parametric analyses may be inaccurate. If the data are skewed to the right, the mean will be an over-estimate of the median value, and if the data are skewed to the left, the mean will be an under-estimate of the median value. However, it is often difficult to estimate whether the significance of the difference between two groups will have been under-estimated or over-estimated as a result of skewness in the data.

Confidence intervals

The 95 per cent confidence interval is an estimate of the range in which there is a 95 per cent probability that the true summary statistic lies and, as such, indicates the precision with which the summary statistic has been measured. The 95 per cent confidence interval should not be confused with the interval defined by the mean $\pm$ 2 SDs. The interval defined by the mean $\pm$ 2 SDs is the range in which 95 per cent of the data points lie. The 95 per cent confidence interval, which is an estimate of precision, complements the information obtained by summary statistics such as estimates of incidence, prevalence, mean values, odds ratios etc., and can easily be calculated using a statistical computer program or the computer program CIA.[7]

When comparing summary statistics between two or more groups, the extent to which the confidence intervals overlap indicates whether there are any statistically significant differences between groups. Some simple rules that can be applied to confidence intervals are shown in Table 6.4. An explanation of how the extent of the overlap reflects the P value is shown in Example 6.2. These rules can be applied to many summary statistics such as prevalence rates, mean values, mean differences and odds ratios.

Table 6.4   Visual interpretation of confidence intervals for summary statistics such as prevalence or incidence rates, mean values, odds ratios etc.

Relative position of confidence intervals	Statistical significance between groups
Do not overlap	Highly significant difference
Overlap, but one summary statistic is not within the confidence interval for the other	Possibly significant, but not highly
Overlap and one summary statistic is within the interval for the other	Probably not significant
Overlap to a large extent	Definitely not significant

Health science research

Figure 6.5   Interpretation of the overlap of the 95% confidence intervals
in three study groups

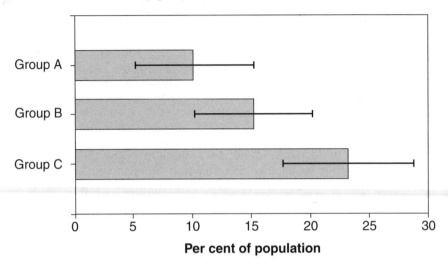

Example 6.2   Interpretation of overlap of confidence intervals

Group A vs C P=0.002
Group A vs B P=0.402
Group B vs C P=0.048

An example of the relation between the overlap of 95% confidence
intervals and P values is shown in Figure 6.5. From the figure, it can be
seen that the incidence rates in groups A and C are significantly different
because the 95% confidence intervals for the two groups do not overlap.
This confirms the P value of 0.002 for the difference between groups A
and C.

Similarly, it can be seen that the incidence rates in groups A and B
are not significantly different because the 95% confidence intervals
overlap and the incidence in group B is with the upper interval of
group A. This confirms the P value of 0.402 for the difference between
groups A and B.

However, the incidence rate in group C is not within the upper interval
for group B and the 95% confidence intervals overlap to a small extent.
This confirms the P value of 0.048 for the difference between groups B
and C, which is of marginal significance.

Baseline comparisons

In many studies, the first analysis is usually to compare the characteristics of the subjects in each group in order to estimate whether important confounders are evenly balanced between the study groups or whether there are any important biases that may explain the results. In randomised trials, the randomisation procedures should ensure that characteristics are quite evenly balanced between the study groups but in other studies such as non-randomised trials, small trials or case-control studies, further statistical methods may be needed to reduce the effects that can result from an imbalance of confounders.

When reporting the baseline characteristics of continuously distributed variables, it is important that information of the mean and its standard deviation is given. The standard error and the closely related 95 per cent confidence interval are not appropriate statistics to use in this situation because they are estimates of precision.[8] When comparing baseline characteristics, we are actually interested in whether the spread of the data is comparable in the study groups, not whether we have estimated the mean value of each characteristic with precision.

Similarly, significance tests are not a valid method with which to assess whether the groups are comparable. Statistical significance depends on many features of the data including the sample size, the size of the standard deviation and the number of tests conducted. If twenty characteristics were compared with significance tests, we would expect that one of the tests would be significant at the $P<0.05$ level merely by chance variation. Rather than using statistical tests, the absolute differences in baseline characteristics between groups are better judged in terms of their clinical importance, prior knowledge of their effects and their ability to influence the outcomes of the study. Any differences that are judged to be important, regardless of statistical significance, should be adjusted for using multivariate analyses such as multiple or logistic regression.[9] If no important differences are evident, then the data analyses are usually a quite simple comparison of outcomes between study groups.

Table 6.5 shows the baseline characteristics of four study groups enrolled in a randomised controlled trial.[10] The authors have correctly reported the number of each gender in each group and the means of other baseline characteristics without performing any significance tests. However, in this study, the standard deviations are not a good description of the spread of the data of age and duration of illness because a quick calculation of the mean ± 2 standard deviations gives a range that includes negative values for both variables. In this study, the data for these variables are skewed and therefore the median age and duration of illness with the inter-quartile range would have been more accurate statistics with which to describe the baseline characteristics.

Table 6.5 Baseline characteristics of study groups in the double-blind randomised controlled trial shown in Example 2.1 in Chapter 2[11]

Characteristic	Placebo group 1 N=49	Placebo group 2 N=49	Active group 1 N=51	Active group 2 N=51
Gender				
Male	21	24	29	31
Female	28	25	22	20
Age in months (mean ± SD) (range)	14.0 + 14.3 (2–71)	17.8 ± 29.0 (2–187)	15.1 ± 10.4 (2–52)	15.2 ± 12.3 (2–62)
Duration of illness before admission (hr) (mean ± SD)	34 ± 21	42 ± 26	35 ± 30	55 ± 42

Bivariate and multivariate methods

Once the research question has been framed, the distribution of each variable is evident, the variables have been categorised into outcome, intervening or explanatory variables (Chapter 3) and the baseline characteristics have been investigated, the statistical analyses are usually quite straightforward. Table 6.6 shows how to use the flowcharts shown in Figures 6.6 to 6.8 that provide a guide to selecting the correct statistical analysis for the data set being analysed.

Table 6.6 Guide to statistical decision flowcharts

Condition	Figure
One outcome variable	Figure 6.6
Two variables	Figure 6.7
More than two variables	Figure 6.8

When selecting a statistical method to calculate P values, it may be more informative to also calculate complementary descriptive statistics.[12] For example, if 30 per cent of the control group in a study develop an illness compared to 10 per cent of the intervention group, then it may be more relevant to report this as a risk reduction of 20 per cent rather than to simply compute a chi-square value. The confidence interval around this risk reduction, which will depend on the sample size in each study group, will provide further information of the precision of this estimate. Finally, a graph to demonstrate the size of the difference between any reported statistics will help in the clinical interpretation of the results.

Figure 6.6   Decision flowchart for analyses with only one outcome variable

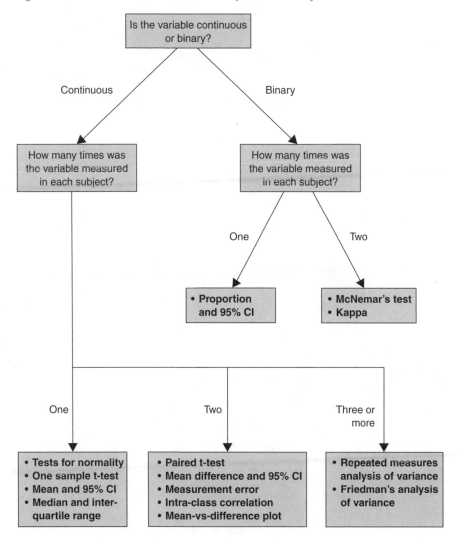

Figure 6.7 Decision flowchart for analyses with two variables

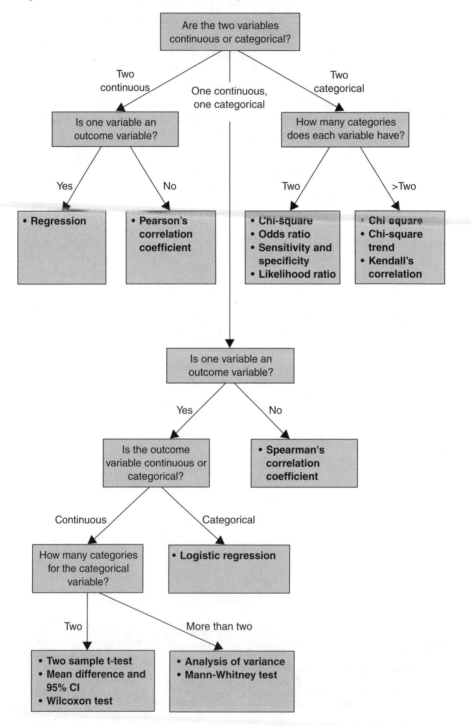

Figure 6.8   Decision flowchart for analyses involving more than two variables

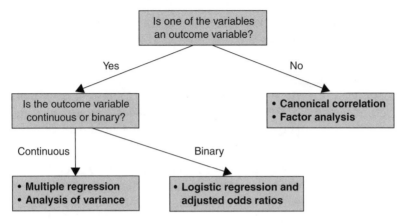

Intention-to-treat analyses

Intention-to-treat analyses are based on maintaining all of the subjects in the groups into which they were initially randomised regardless of any subsequent events or unexpected outcomes. In randomised trials in which intention-to-treat analyses are not used, the clinical effect that a treatment can be expected to have in the general community may be over-estimated.[13]

In intention-to-treat analyses, it is important not to re-categorise subjects according to whether they changed treatment, were non-compliant or dropped out of the study. In essence, intention-to-treat analyses have the effect of maintaining the balance of confounders between groups that the randomisation process ensured. Intention-to-treat analyses also minimise the effects of selection bias caused by subjects who drop out of the study or who are non-compliant with the study treatments.

It is sometimes difficult to include drop-outs in intention-to-treat analyses because the data of their final outcomes are not available. For subjects who do not complete the study, the final data collected from each subject should be included in the intention-to-treat analysis regardless of the follow-up period attained.

The benefits of using intention-to-treat analysis are shown in Table 6.7. Intention-to-treat analyses provide an estimation of the expected effect that a new treatment or intervention will have in a similar sample of patients. However, these types of analyses will almost always under-estimate the absolute effect of the intervention on the study outcome in subjects who are highly compliant. For this reason, intention-to-treat analyses may be

Glossary

Term	Meaning
Intention-to-treat analyses	Analyses based on maintaining all subjects in the analyses in the groups to which they were originally randomised and regardless of dropping out
Restricted or preferred analyses	Analyses limited to compliant subjects only, that is subjects who complete the study and who are known to have maintained the treatment to which they were randomised
As-treated analyses	Analyses in which subjects are re-grouped according to the treatment they actually received, which may not be the treatment to which they were randomised

misleading if the study is badly designed or is conducted in a way that does not maximise compliance.[14] In practice, intention-to-treat analyses are a good estimate of the effectiveness of treatments or interventions in which the effects of bias and confounding have been minimised, but they will almost certainly under-estimate efficacy.

Table 6.7 Features of intention-to-treat analyses
• maintain the balance of confounders achieved by randomisation
• avoid a preferred analysis based on only a subset of subjects
• ensure that subjective decisions about omitting some subjects from the analysis do not cause bias
• minimise the problems of drop-outs and protocol violations
• may require 'last values' being used in the analysis if subjects cannot be followed
• usually under-estimate 'pure' treatment effects and thus are used to measure effectiveness and not efficacy

In some studies, a pragmatic approach may be adopted in which both an intention-to-treat analysis and an 'as-treated' analysis that includes only the subjects who are known to have complied with the protocol are presented. It is appropriate to included *as-treated* analyses, which are sometimes called *per-protocol analyses*, when the condition of the patient changes unexpectedly and it becomes unethical to maintain the treatment to which

they have been allocated. However, analyses by intention-to-treat, by com-
pliers only or using 'as-treated' criteria may provide very different results
from one another and should be interpreted with caution.[15] The process of
adjusting for estimates of compliance using more sophisticated analyses that
take into account compliance information, such as pill counts, can become
complicated. Compliance often fluctuates over time and is rarely an all or
nothing event so that odds ratios of effect in groups of subjects with poor,
moderate and good compliance may need to be compared.[16]

An example of dual reporting is shown in Table 6.8. In studies such as
this, in which the two analyses provide different results, it is important to
recognise that the restricted analysis is likely to be biased, may not be balanced for confounders and will provide an over-optimistic estimate of the
treatment effects than could be attained in practice.

Table 6.8	Results of an intention-to-treat analysis and an analysis restricted to children actually receiving the active treatment in a controlled trail of diazepam to prevent recurrent febrile seizures[17]	
	Reduction of seizures	Relative risk of seizure when treated with diazepam
Intention-to treat analysis	44%	0.56 (95% CI 0.38, 0.81)
Restricted analyses	82%	0.18 (95% CI 0.09, 0.37)

7

REPORTING THE RESULTS

Section 1—Repeatability

The objectives of this section are to understand how to:
- assess the precision of a measurement;
- design a study to measure repeatability;
- estimate various measures of repeatability and understand how they relate to one another;
- estimate repeatability when there are more than two measurements per subject; and
- interpret the results when they are displayed graphically.

Measuring repeatability

In any research study, the accuracy with which the observations have been measured is of fundamental importance. Repeatability is a measure of the consistency of a method and, as such, is the extent to which an instrument produces exactly the same result when it is used in the same subject on more than one occasion. Measurements of repeatability are sometimes referred to as *reproducibility*, *reliability*, *consistency* or *test-retest* variability—these terms are used interchangeably to convey the same meaning.

An instance of a study in which the repeatability of an instrument was measured is shown in Example 7.1. The statistical methods that can be used to assess repeatability are summarised in Table 7.1.

Characteristic	Description
Example 7.1 Study to test repeatability Childs et al. Suprasternal Doppler ultrasound for assessment of stroke distance.[1]	
Aims	To assess the repeatability of Doppler ultrasound measurements for measuring cardiac output (stroke distance) in children
Type of study	Methodology study
Sample base	Healthy primary and pre-school children
Subjects	72 children age 4–11 years
Outcome measurements	Six measurements of stroke distance using Doppler
Explanatory measurements	Heart rate, age, height, weight, gender
Statistics	Measurement error, mean-vs-differences plot
Conclusion	• the stroke distance measurements vary by up to 2 cm • between-operator variation was $\pm$ 5.3 cm • there was a modest correlation between stroke distance and age and heart rate
Strengths	• the order of the operators was randomised • the operators were blinded to the stroke distance value • correct statistical analyses were used
Limitations	• only healthy children were enrolled so the results cannot be extrapolated to children with cardiac problems

Table 7.1	Statistical methods for assessing within-subject, within-observer and between-observer repeatability
Type of data	**Statistical test**
Continuous data	Measurement error
	Paired t-test and Levine's test of equal variance
	Mean difference and 95% confidence interval
	Mean-vs-differences or mean-vs-variance plot
	Intraclass correlation coefficient
Categorical data	Kappa
	Proportion in agreement
	Average correct classification rate

For continuously distributed measurements, repeatability is best assessed using both the measurement error and the intraclass correlation coefficient (ICC) to give an indication of how much reliance can be placed on a single measurement. In addition, a mean-vs-differences plot, or a mean-vs-variance plot for when more than two repeated measurements are taken, can be used to estimate the absolute consistency of the method or whether there is any systematic bias between measurements taken for example on different days or by two different observers.[2]

Measurement error is used to assess the absolute range in which a subject's 'true' measurement can be expected to lie. For continuous measurements, measurement error is often called the standard error of the measurement (SEM) or described as Sw. To complement the information provided by estimates of the measurement error, ICC is used to assess relative consistency and a mean-vs-differences or mean-vs-variance plot is used to assess the absolute consistency of the measurements and the extent of any systematic bias.

For categorical measurements, repeatability is often called *misclassification error* and can be assessed using kappa, the proportion in agreement and the average correct classification rate.

When assessing the repeatability of either continuous or categorical measurements, we recommend that the full range of repeatability statistics shown in Table 7.1 is computed because the calculation of one statistic in the absence of the others is difficult to interpret.

Repeatability of continuous measurements

Variation in a measurement made using the same instrument to test the same subject on different occasions can arise from any one of the four sources shown in Table 7.2.

| Table 7.2 | Sources of variation in measurements |

- within-observer variation (intra-observer error)
- between-observer variation (inter-observer error)
- within-subject variations (test-retest error)
- changes in the subject following an intervention (responsiveness)

Within-observer variation may arise from inconsistent measurement practices on the part of the observer, from equipment variation or from variations in the ways in which observers interpret results. Similarly, within-subject variations may arise from variations in subject compliance with the testing procedure, or from biological or equipment variations. These sources of variation from the observer, the subject, and the equipment prevent us from estimating the 'true' value of a measurement. The two statistics that can be used to estimate the magnitude of these sources of variation are the measurement error, which is an absolute estimate of repeatability, and the ICC, which is a relative estimate of repeatability. The interpretation of these statistics is shown in Table 7.3 and the methods for calculating these statistics are described in detail below.

| Table 7.3 | Methods of describing repeatability such as within-observer, between-observer and between-day variations in measurements |

Measurement	Interpretation
Measurement error	Measure of the within-subject test-retest variation—sometimes called the standard error of the measurement (SEM)
95% range	Range in which there is 95% certainty that the 'true' value for a subject lies—sometimes called the 'limits of agreement'
Mean-vs-differences or mean-vs-variance plot	Plot used to demonstrate absolute repeatability and to investigate whether the test-retest error is systematic or random across the entire range of measurements
Intraclass correlation coefficient	Ratio of the between-subject variance to the total variance for continuous measurements—a value of 1 indicates perfect repeatability because no within-subject variance would be present

Cont'd

Table 7.3 Cont'd   Methods of describing repeatability such as within-observer, between-observer and between-day variations in measurements

Measurement	Interpretation
Paired t-test, mean difference and 95% confidence interval	Statistical method to test whether the test-retest variation is of a significant magnitude and to describe the average magnitude of the test-retest differences
Levine's test of equal variance	Statistical method to test whether there is a significant difference in repeatability between two different study groups
Kappa	A statistic similar to ICC that is used for categorical measurements—a value of 1 indicates perfect agreement
Proportion in agreement and average correct classification rate	Measurements used to describe the absolute repeatablility for categorical measurements

The ICC is a relative estimate of repeatability because it is an estimate of the proportion of the total variance that is accounted for by the variation between subjects. The remaining variance can then be attributed to the variation between repeated measurements within subjects. Thus, a high ICC indicates that only a small proportion of the variance can be attributed to within-subject differences. In contrast, the measurement error gives an estimate of the absolute range in which the 'true' value for a subject is expected to lie.

When we test a subject, we hope to obtain the 'true' value of a measurement but factors such as subject compliance and equipment errors result in variation around the true estimate. The amount of measurement error attributable to these sources can be estimated from the variation, or standard deviation, around duplicate or triplicate measurements taken from the same subjects.

The study design for measuring repeatability was discussed in Chapter 2. Basically, repeatability is estimated by taking multiple measurements from a group of subjects. It is common to take only two measurements from each subject although a greater number, such as triplicate or quadruple measurements, gives a more precise estimate and can be used to increase precision when the number of subjects is limited.

Influence of selection bias

Because both the measurement error and the ICC are influenced by selection bias, the unqualified repeatability of a test cannot be estimated. The measurements of ICC and measurement error calculated from any study are only applicable to the situation in which they are estimated and cannot be compared between studies in which methods such as the subject selection criteria are different.

Estimates of ICC tend to be higher and measurement error tends to be lower (that is both indicate that the instrument is more precise) in studies in which there is more variation in the sample as a result of the inclusion criteria.[3] This occurs because the between-subject variation is larger for the same within-subject variation, that is the denominator is larger for the same numerator. For this reason, measurements of ICC will be higher in studies in which subjects are selected randomly from a population or in which subjects with a wide range of measurements are deliberately selected. Conversely, for the same instrument, measurements of ICC will be lower in studies in which measurements are only collected from clinic attenders who have a narrower range of values that are at the more severe end of the measurement scale.

In addition, estimates of measurement error and ICC from studies in which three or four repeated measurements have been taken cannot be compared directly with estimates from studies in which only two repeated measurements are used. Such comparisons are invalid because a larger number of repeat measurements from each subject gives a more precise estimate of repeatability.

Sample size requirements

The sample size that is required to measure repeatability is discussed in Chapter 4. To calculate ICC, a minimum of 30 subjects is needed to ensure that the variance can be correctly estimated. Of course, a sample size of 60–70 subjects will give a more precise estimate, but a sample larger than 100 subjects is rarely required.

Measurement error calculated from two measurements per subject

To establish the measurement error attributable to within-subject variation, analyses based on paired data must be used. For this, the mean difference between the two measurements and the standard deviation of the differences has to be calculated. The measurement error can then be calculated by dividing the standard deviation of the differences by the square root of 2, that is the number of measurements per subject,[4] i.e.:

$$\text{Measurement error} = \text{SD of differences} / \sqrt{2}$$

Table 7.4 shows measurements of weight in 30 subjects studied on two separate occasions. The four columns of the differences, differences squared, sum and mean are used for calculations of repeatability and ICC that are described later in this section. From the table, the mean difference between the weights measured on two occasions is 0.22 kg and the standard deviation of the differences is 1.33 kg. From the equation shown above:

$$\text{Measurement error} = \text{SD of differences} / \sqrt{2}$$
$$= 1.33 / 1.414$$
$$= 0.94 \text{ kg}$$

Table 7.4   Weight measured in 30 subjects on two different occasions

Number	Time 1	Time 2	Difference	Difference^2	Sum	Mean
1	50.0	51.6	1.6	2.6	101.6	50.8
2	58.0	57.9	−0.1	0.0	115.9	58.0
3	47.7	50.9	3.2	10.2	98.6	49.3
4	43.6	42.9	−0.7	0.5	86.5	43.3
5	41.1	41.9	0.8	0.6	83.0	41.5
6	54.6	55.4	0.8	0.6	110.0	55.0
7	48.6	47.3	−1.3	1.7	95.9	48.0
8	56.2	55.5	−0.7	0.5	111.7	55.9
9	56.0	55.4	−0.6	0.4	111.4	55.7
10	41.8	39.8	−2.0	4.0	81.6	40.8
11	51.5	52.4	0.9	0.8	103.9	52.0
12	49.2	51.0	1.8	3.2	100.2	50.1
13	54.5	54.9	0.4	0.2	109.4	54.7
14	46.8	45.5	−1.3	1.7	92.3	46.2
15	44.7	45.0	0.3	0.1	89.7	44.9
16	58.0	59.9	1.9	3.6	117.9	59.0
17	54.0	53.9	−0.1	0.0	107.9	54.0
18	47.5	47.2	−0.3	0.1	94.7	47.4
19	45.3	45.2	−0.1	0.0	90.5	45.3
20	47.5	50.6	3.1	9.6	98.1	49.1

Cont'd

Table 7.4 Cont'd   Weight measured in 30 subjects on two different
occasions

Number	Time 1	Time 2	Difference	Difference²	Sum	Mean
21	44.7	44.0	−0.7	0.5	88.7	44.4
22	52.9	52.2	−0.7	0.5	105.1	52.6
23	53.8	52.9	−0.9	0.8	106.7	53.4
24	44.9	45.2	0.3	0.1	90.1	45.1
25	47.5	49.9	2.4	5.8	97.4	48.7
26	49.3	47.4	−1.9	3.6	96.7	48.4
27	45.0	44.9	−0.1	0.0	89.9	45.0
28	62.4	61.7	−0.7	0.5	124.1	62.1
29	46.4	47.1	0.7	0.5	93.5	46.8
30	52.0	52.6	0.6	0.4	104.6	52.3
Sum	1495.50	1502.10	6.60	53.04	2997.60	—
Mean	49.85	50.07	0.22	1.77	99.92	—
Variance	27.90	29.63	1.78	7.08	113.07	—
SD	5.28	5.44	1.33	2.66	10.64	—

The measurement error can then be converted into a 95 per cent range using the formula:

$$95\% \text{ range} = \text{Measurement error} \times t$$

Note that, for this calculation, t is not determined by the study sample size because a confidence interval is not being computed around the sample mean. In this calculation, a value for t of 1.96 is used as a critical value to estimate the 95 per cent range for an individual 'true' value. Thus:

$$
\begin{aligned}
95\% \text{ range} &= \text{Measurement error} \times t \\
&= (\text{SD of differences} / \sqrt{2}) \times t \\
&= (1.33 / 1.414) \times 1.96 \\
&= 0.94 \times 1.96 \\
&= 1.85 \text{ kg}
\end{aligned}
$$

This value indicates that the 'true' value for 95 per cent of the subjects lies within this range above and below the value of actual measurement taken. In practice, there is no way of knowing whether the first or the second measurement taken from a subject is nearer to their 'true' value because it is impossible to know what the 'true' value is. However, for a subject whose weight was measured as 60.0 kg, we can say that we would be 95 per cent certain that the subject's 'true' value lies within the range 60 ± 1.85 kg; that is, between 58.15 and 61.85 kg.

Use of paired t-tests

From Table 7.4, we can see that the mean difference between the time 1 and time 2 measurements is 0.22 kg with a standard deviation of 1.33 kg. The 95 per cent confidence interval around this difference, calculated using a computer program, is an interval of −0.24 to 0.68 kg. Because this encompasses the zero value of no difference, it confirms that the two measurements are not significantly different. In practice, this is not surprising since we would not expect to find a significant difference between two measurements made in the same people on two different occasions.

A problem with using a paired t-test to describe repeatability is that large positive within-subject differences are balanced by large negative within-subject differences. Thus, this statistic tends to 'hide' large errors such as the four subjects in Table 7.4 who had a difference of 2 kg or greater between days of measurements. However, t-tests are useful for assessing the extent of any systematic bias between observers or over time and the confidence interval around the mean difference provides an estimate of the precision of the difference that has been measured.

Comparing repeatability between two groups

A test of equal variance can be useful for comparing the repeatability of a measurement between two separate groups of subjects. For example, we may have measured the repeatability of pain scores in two groups of subjects, that is one group of surgical patients and one group of non-surgical patients. To judge whether the scores are more repeatable in one group than the other, we could calculate the mean difference in scores for each patient in each group, and then compare the variance around the mean difference in each group using Levine's test of equal variances. Some computer package programs calculate this statistic in the procedure for an unpaired t-test.

A significant result from Levine's test would indicate that the standard deviation around the mean differences is significantly lower in one group than the other, and therefore that the test is more repeatable in that group. Calculation of the measurement error for each group will also give us a good idea of the difference in the absolute repeatability of the pain scores in each group.

Mean-vs-differences plot

A plot of the mean value against the difference between measurements for each subject that are shown in Table 7.4 can be used to determine whether the measurement error is related to the size of the measurement. This type of plot is called a mean-vs-differences plot or a 'Bland & Altman' plot after the statisticians who first reported its merit in repeatability applications.[5] The mean-vs-differences data from Table 7.4 are plotted in Figure 7.1. This plot gives an impression of the absolute differences between measurements that are not so obvious in the scatter plot of the same data. A scatter plot is shown in Figure 7.2 but this is not a good method with which to describe repeatability.

Figure 7.1   Mean-vs-differences plot

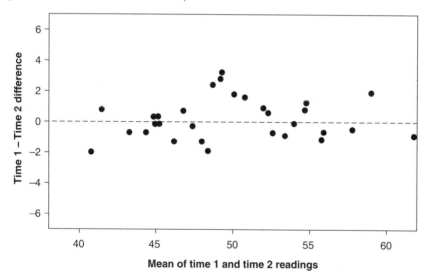

Mean of time 1 and time 2 readings

A mean-vs-differences plot of readings taken on two separate occasions from the same group of subjects in order to estimate the repeatability of the measurements.

A rank correlation coefficient for the mean-vs-differences plot, called Kendall's correlation coefficient, can be used to assess whether the differences are related to the size of the measurement. For the data shown in Figure 7.1, Kendall's tau b = 0.07 with P=0.6, which confirms the lack of any statistically significant systematic bias.

Health science research

The shape of the scatter in the means-vs-differences plot conveys a great deal of information about the repeatability of the measurements. To examine the scatter, we recommend that the total length of the y-axis represent one-third to one-half of the length of the x-axis. The interpretation of the shape of the scatter is shown in Table 7.5. Clearly, measurements that are highly repeatable with only a small amount of random error, as indicated by a narrow scatter around the line of no difference, will provide far more accurate data than measurements that are less repeatable or that have a systematic error. Obviously, a scatter that is above or below the line of zero difference would indicate that there is a systematic bias. This is easily adjusted for in the situation in which it is measured, but ultimately detracts from the repeatability of the instrument because the extent of the error will not be known for situations in which it has not been measured, and therefore cannot be adjusted for.

Figure 7.2   Scatter plot

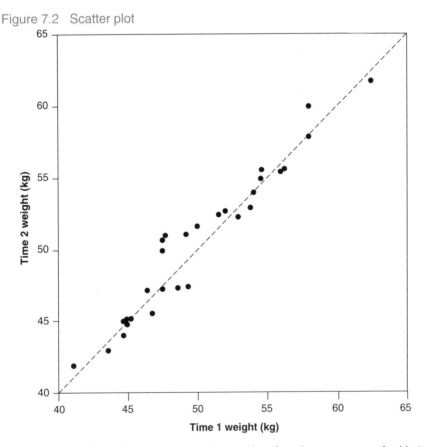

Scatter plot of readings taken on two separate occasions from the same group of subjects shown with line of identity.

Table 7.5	Interpretation of mean-vs-differences plots	
Example	Shape of scatter	Interpretation
Figure 7.3	Close to line of zero difference	Measurement is repeatable and the error is random
Figure 7.4	Wide scatter around line of zero difference	Measurement is not repeatable but the error is random
Figure 7.5	Funnel shaped	Measurement is quite repeatable at the lower end of the scale but increases as the measurement increases, i.e. is related to the size of the measurement
Figure 7.6	Scatter is not parallel to line of zero difference	The error is not constant along the entire scale indicating a systematic bias

Figure 7.3 Mean-vs-differences plot

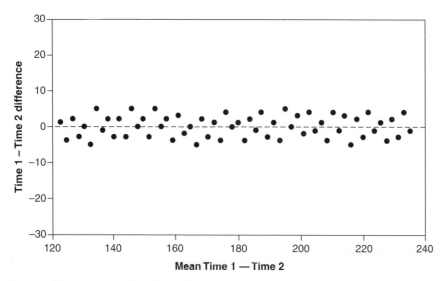

Mean-vs-differences plot of readings taken on two separate occasions from the same group of subjects showing that there is good repeatability between the measurements as indicated by a narrow scatter around the zero line of no difference.

Health science research

Figure 7.4   Mean-vs-differences plot

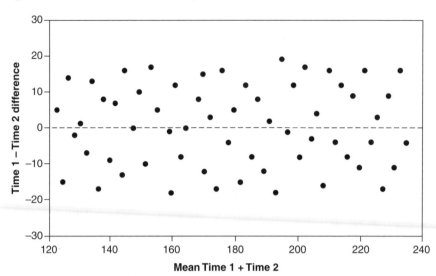

Mean-vs-differences plot of readings taken on two separate occasions from the same group of subjects showing that there is poor repeatability between the measurements as indicated by a wide scatter around the zero line of no difference.

Figure 7.5   Mean-vs-differences plot

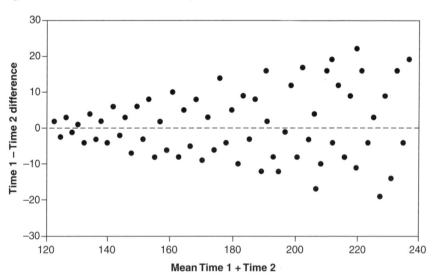

Mean-vs-differences plot of readings taken on two separate occasions from the same group of subjects showing that there is a systematic error in the repeatability between the measurements as indicated by a funnel shaped scatter around the zero line of no difference.

Figure 7.6   Mean-vs-differences plot

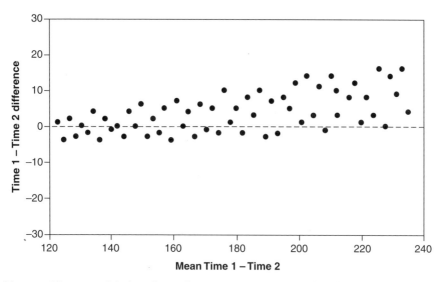

Mean-vs-differences plot of readings taken on two separate occasions from the same group of subjects showing that there is good repeatability between the measurements at the lower end of the scale but a bias that increases towards the higher end of the measurement scale.

Measurement error calculated from more than two measurements per subject

If more than two measurements are taken for each subject, as shown in Table 7.6, the measurement error is calculated slightly differently. Firstly, the variance is calculated for each subject and from this, the mean of the variances for each subject (the within-subject variances) can be derived. From the example data shown in Table 7.6 in which four measurements were taken from each subject, the mean within-subject variance is 1.42. The square root of the mean variance is then used to estimate the measurement error as follows:

$$
\begin{aligned}
\text{Measurement error} &= S_w \\
&= \sqrt{\text{mean within-subject variance}} \\
&= \sqrt{1.42} \\
&= 1.19
\end{aligned}
$$

The measurement error expressed as a 95 per cent range is then as follows:

$$
\begin{aligned}
95\% \text{ range} &= \pm \text{ Measurement error} \times t \\
&= \pm 1.19 \times 1.96 \\
&= \pm 2.34 \text{ kg.}
\end{aligned}
$$

Health science research

This is slightly wider than the estimate of a 95 per cent range of ± 1.85 kg calculated from two measurements per subject as in the example from the data shown in Table 7.4. The larger value is a result of the larger number of measurements per subject, which leads to a wider variation in the mean values for each subject. However, this is a more precise estimate of the measurement error.

Table 7.6		Weight measured in 30 adults on four different occasions				
Number	Time 1	Time 2	Time 3	Time 4	Mean	Variance
1	50.0	51.6	50.0	52.1	50.9	1.18
2	58.0	57.9	58.7	59.1	58.4	0.33
3	47.7	50.9	50.9	49.1	49.7	2.41
4	43.6	42.0	44.8	42.8	43.5	0.85
5	41.1	41.9	41.5	43.2	41.9	0.83
6	54.6	55.4	56.3	55.4	55.4	0.48
7	48.6	47.3	49.7	46.5	48.0	2.00
8	56.2	55.5	57.4	58.5	56.9	1.75
9	56.0	55.4	56.9	56.5	56.2	0.42
10	41.8	39.8	42.0	40.1	40.9	1.29
11	51.5	52.4	50.1	52.3	51.6	1.13
12	49.2	51.0	52.0	49.5	50.4	1.72
13	54.5	54.9	55.8	55.2	55.1	0.30
14	46.8	45.5	46.4	48.5	46.8	1.58
15	44.7	45.0	46.8	44.2	45.2	1.28
16	58.0	59.9	59.2	59.8	59.2	0.76
17	54.0	53.9	54.7	51.8	53.6	1.57
18	47.5	47.2	49.7	46.9	47.8	1.62
19	45.3	45.2	46.3	48.1	46.2	1.81
20	47.5	50.6	49.1	51.3	49.6	2.85
21	44.7	44.0	46.3	43.7	44.7	1.35
22	52.9	52.2	53.9	50.6	52.4	1.93
23	53.8	52.9	51.3	53.4	52.9	1.20
24	44.9	45.2	48.0	45.6	45.9	2.00

Cont'd

Table 7.6 Cont'd Weight measured in 30 adults on four different occasions

Number	Time 1	Time 2	Time 3	Time 4	Mean	Variance
25	47.5	49.9	48.6	51.2	49.3	2.57
26	49.3	47.4	47.9	50.8	48.9	2.34
27	45.0	44.9	47.4	44.4	45.4	1.80
28	62.4	61.7	61.4	61.7	61.8	0.18
29	46.4	47.1	46.9	49.4	47.5	1.78
30	52.0	52.6	52.7	50.2	51.9	1.34
Mean	49.9	50.1	50.8	50.4	50.3	1.42

The mean within-subject variance for the data shown in Table 7.6 can also be estimated using a one-way analysis of variance (ANOVA) with the 'subjects' assigned as the 'group' variable. In this case, a table or a spreadsheet with a different format from that shown in Table 7.6 would be needed. To perform the ANOVA, the four values for each subject would have to be represented on separate data lines but with the data for each subject identified with a unique identification number that is used as the 'group' variable in the analysis. Thus, for the data above, the number of 'cases' would become 120 with 119 degrees of freedom and the number of 'groups' would be 30 with 29 degrees of freedom. The one-way analysis of variance table for these data is shown in Table 7.7.

Table 7.7 One-way analysis of variance for data shown in Table 7.6

	Degrees of freedom	Sum of squares	Mean square	Variance ratio (F)	P
Subjects	29	3155.5	108.8	76.55	<0.0001
Residual	90	127.9	1.42		
Total	119	3283.5			

As can be seen, the mean square of the residuals is 1.42, which is the same number as the mean variance calculated in Table 7.6.

When more than two measurements are taken, a mean-vs-standard deviations plot, which is shown in Figure 7.7, can be used to check for a systematic relation between the differences as indicated by the standard deviation for each subject and the size of the measurement. Again, a rank correlation coefficient can be used to investigate whether a systematic error exists. For the data shown in Figure 7.7, Kendall's tau b is -0.19 with $P=0.13$ which confirms the absence of systematic bias.

Figure 7.7 Mean-vs-standard deviations plot

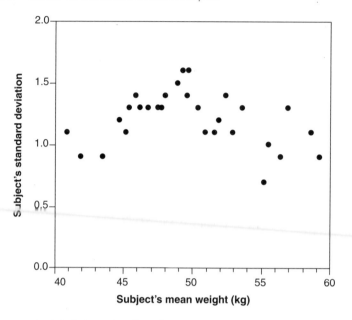

A mean-vs-standard deviations plot of readings taken on four separate occasions from the same group of subjects in order to estimate the repeatability of the measurements.

Interpretation

An estimate of measurement error that is small indicates that the method of obtaining a measurement is reliable, or consistent. However, a measurement error that is large indicates that a single measurement is an unreliable estimate of the 'true' value for the subject. This is a problem if the instrument has to be used in a research project because no better alternative is available. In this case, several measurements may need to be taken from each subject and a decision to use the highest, the lowest or the mean will need to be made, depending on a consensus decision of people who are expert in interpreting measurements from the equipment.

In clinical studies, the measurement error around a subject's readings taken at baseline can be regarded as the range in which 'normal' values for that particular subject can be expected to lie. If the subject has an outcome measurement at a later study or following an intervention that lies outside their own estimated 'normal' range, they can be regarded as having an 'abnormal' response; that is, a measurement that has significantly improved or significantly decreased from baseline. This approach is much the same as regarding the result of a screening test as 'abnormal' if a measurement is less than 1.96 standard deviations below the mean for normal subjects. This approach is also similar to regarding an intervention as successful if an individual subject improves from the 'abnormal' range into the 'normal' range for the population.

Intraclass correlation coefficient

The ICC is used to describe the extent to which multiple measurements taken from the same subject are related. This correlation, which is a measure of the proportion of the variance in within-subject measurements that can be attributed to 'true' differences between subjects, is often called a *reliability coefficient*. The ICC is calculated from the ratio of the variance between subjects to the total variance, which is comprised of both the subjects' variance plus the error variance. Thus, a high ICC value such as 0.9 indicates that 90 per cent of the variance is due to 'true' variance between subjects and 10 per cent is due to measurement error, or within-subject variance.

The advantage of the ICC is that, unlike Pearson's correlation, a value of unity is obtained only when the values for the two measurements are identical to one another. Thus, if either a random or systematic difference occurs, the ICC is reduced. Unlike other correlation coefficients, the ICC does not have to be squared to interpret the percentage of the variation explained.

Calculating the ICC is particularly appropriate when the order of the measurements has no meaning, for example when subjects undergo each of two methods in random order or when the error between different observers using the same method (inter-rater agreement) is being estimated. However, there are different methods for calculating ICC that depend on the selection of the study sample.

Care must be taken when selecting the type of ICC calculation that is used because the results can be quite different.[6] Few computer programs estimate ICC directly but values can be fairly easily calculated manually from an analysis of variance table. Three methods of calculation are shown below that either include or exclude observer bias. Two of the methods make different assumptions about the observers and the third method is a simplified formula that can be used when only two measurements are taken for each subject.

Method 1

This method is used when the difference between observers is fixed, that is the proportion of measurements taken by each observer does not change. For this method, a one-way analysis of variance table is used. This ICC is appropriate for studies in which the same observers are always used. There are small variations in the calculation of this ICC in the literature but the different calculations all give similar results, especially when the number of subjects is large.

Table 7.8	One-way analysis of variance for data shown in Table 7.4				
	Degrees of freedom	Sum of squares	Mean square	Variance ratio (F)	P
Subjects	29	1642.4	56.64	64.07	<0.0001
Residual	30	26.5	0.88		
Total	59	1668.9			

Using the data shown in Table 7.4, a one-way analysis of variance table as shown in Table 7.8 can be computed. To calculate this table, a table or spreadsheet with the readings from each day for each subject on separate lines is required, and each subject needs an identification number which is used as the 'group' variable. Thus, there will be 60 lines in the file. From the analysis of variance table, the calculation of ICC is as follows.[7] In the calculation, m is the number of repeated measurements and SS is the sum of squares as calculated in the analysis of variance:

$$ICC = \frac{(m \times \text{Between subjects SS}) - \text{Total SS}}{(m-1) \times \text{Total SS}}$$

$$= \frac{(2 \times 1642.4) - 1668.9}{1 \times 1668.9}$$

$$= 0.984$$

The interpretation of this coefficient is that 98.4 per cent of the variance in weight results from the 'true' variance between subjects and that 1.6 per cent can be attributed to the measurement error associated with the equipment used.

If the data from Table 7.6 with four readings a subject was used and the values were substituted into the equation above, then ICC can be computed from the analysis of variance table shown in Table 7.7 as follows:

$$ICC = \frac{(4 \times 3155.5 - 3283.5)}{3 \times 3283.5}$$

$$= 0.948$$

The interpretation of this coefficient is that 94.8 per cent of the variance in weight estimation results from the 'true' variance between subjects and that 5.2 per cent can be attributed to the method of measurement. This value is quite close to that calculated from two repeat readings per subject, but is more accurate as a result of the study design in which four measurements per subject rather than two measurements per subject were obtained.

Method 2

This method is used when it is important to include the random effects that result from a study having a number of different observers. In this case, the ICC is calculated using a two-way analysis of variance with the variance partitioned between the subjects, the method and the residual error. The error is then attributed to the variability of the subjects, to systematic errors due to equipment and observer differences, and to the amount of random variation.

The two-way analysis of variance table for the data in Table 7.6 is shown in Table 7.9. Again, to obtain the analysis of variance table, a table or spreadsheet in a different format from that shown in Table 7.6 is required. The spreadsheet will have three columns to indicate subject number, day and reading so that for 30 subjects with four measurements each there will be 120 rows.

Table 7.9	Two-way analysis of variance for data shown in Table 7.6				
	Degrees of freedom	Sum of squares	Mean square	Variance ratio (F)	P
Subjects	29	3155.5	108.8	75.69	<0.0001
Days	3	14.08	4.69		
Residual	87	113.9	1.31		
Total	119	3283.5			

The calculation is then as follows where MS is the mean square. Using common notation, the bracketed terms are calculated first, followed by the product terms and finally the sums and differences. The calculation is as follows in which m is the number of days and N is the number of subjects:

$$ICC = \frac{\text{Subjects MS} - \text{Residual MS}}{\text{Subjects MS} + (m-1) \times \text{Residual MS} + m/N \times (\text{Days MS} - \text{Residual MS})}$$

$$= \frac{108.8 - 1.31}{108.8 + (4-1) \times 1.31 + 4/30 \,(4.69 - 1.31)}$$

$$= \frac{107.49}{108.8 + 3.93 + 0.45}$$

$$= 107.49 / 113.18$$

$$= 0.950$$

Method 3

A simplified formula is available for estimating ICC when only two measurements are available for each subject.[8] This formula is based on the variance of the sums and differences that are shown at the base of Table 7.4. As above, the bracketed terms are calculated first followed by the product terms and finally the sums and differences.

$$ICC = \frac{\text{Sum variance} - \text{Differences variance}}{\text{Sum variance} + \text{Differences variance} + 2/N \times ((N \times \text{Mean difference}^2) - \text{Differences variance})}$$

For the data in Table 7.4:

$$ICC = \frac{113.07 - 1.78}{113.07 + 1.78 + 2/30\,(30 \times (0.22)^2 - 1.78)}$$

$$= \frac{111.29}{113.07 + 1.78 - 0.33}$$

$$= 111.29 \,/\, 114.52$$

$$= 0.972$$

P values and confidence intervals

It is possible to calculate a P value for the ICC. However, measurements in the same subjects, that are taken in order to measure repeatability and agreement, are highly related by nature and the test of significance is generally of no importance. To test if the ICC is significantly different from zero, an F test can be used. The test statistic is F, which is computed as subjects MS/residual MS, with the mean square values from the analysis of variance table being used. The F value has the usual $(N-1)$ and $(N-1) \times (m-1)$ degrees of freedom. The methods for calculating confidence intervals for ICC are somewhat complicated but have been described.[9, 10]

Relation between measurement error and ICC

Although measurement error and ICC are related measures, they do not convey the same information. The approximate mathematical relationship between the measurement error and the ICC for estimating the repeatability of an instrument is as follows:

$$\text{Measurement error} = \text{Total SD} \times \sqrt{1 - ICC}$$

or

$$ICC = 1 - \left[\frac{\text{Measurement error}}{\text{Total SD}}\right]^2$$

where the total SD is the standard deviation that describes the variation between all of the measurements in the data set. This relationship is plotted in Figure 7.8.

Figure 7.8   Standard error of mean and intraclass correlation

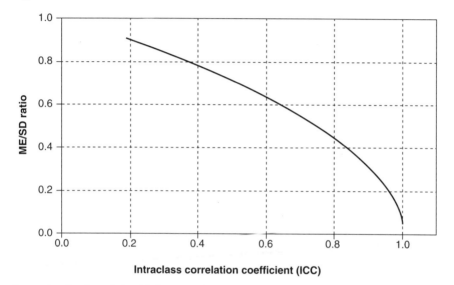

Intraclass correlation coefficient (ICC)

Curve showing the relationship between the measurement error (ME)/standard deviation ratio and the intraclass correlation coefficient.

The formula above shows that ICC is a relative measure of repeatability that relies on the ratio of the measurement error to the total standard deviation. However, measurement error is an absolute term that is positively related to the total standard deviation. These two statistics give very different types of information that complement each other and should be reported together.

It is important to note that, for measurements for which the ICC is reasonably high, say above 0.8, there may still be quite a substantial amount of measurement error. For example, the ICC for Table 7.4 is 0.967 even though four subjects had differences in weights of 2 kg or larger. If the ICC is 0.8, then from the formula above we can calculate that the measurement error is 0.45 standard deviations. This translation from measurement error to ICC can be interpolated from Figure 7.8.

Inappropriate use of Pearson's correlation coefficient and coefficient of variation

The inappropriate use of Pearson's correlation coefficient (R) to describe repeatability or agreement between two methods has been widely discussed in the literature. This coefficient is inappropriate because a perfect corre-lation of one would be found if there was a systematic difference between occasions, for example if the second set of measurements was twice as large as the first. In this case, the repeatability between measurements would be very poor but the correlation would be perfect. A perfect correlation could also be obtained if the regression line through the points deviates from the line of identity.

In practice, Pearson's R is usually higher than the ICC but if the predominant source of error is random, then values computed for Pearson's R and for the ICC will be very close. In any case, the closeness of the two numbers is not of interest since each has a different inter-pretation. Moreover, consideration of Pearson's R is irrelevant because any two measurements that are taken from the same subject will always be closely related.

Coefficient of variation

It is always better to use the ICC than the coefficient of variation, which is the within-subject standard deviation divided by the mean of the meas-urements. The interpretation of the coefficient of variation is as a percentage, that is a coefficient of 0.045 is interpreted as 4.5 per cent. However, this figure implies that there is a systematic error even in data sets in which no such bias exists because 4.5 per cent of the lowest meas-urement in the data set is much smaller than 4.5 per cent of the highest measurement. In addition, coefficients of variation can clearly only ever be compared between study samples in which the means of the measurements are identical.

Repeatability of categorical data

The repeatability of categorical data such as the presence of exposures or illnesses or other types of information collected by questionnaires can also be estimated. In such situations, the measurement error is usually called *misclassification error*. The conditions under which the repeatability of questionnaires can be measured are shown in Table 7.10. If a questionnaire is to be used in a community setting, then repeatability has to be established in a similar community setting and not in specific samples such as clinic attenders, who form a well-defined subsample of a population. Also, the repeatability of an instrument should not be established in patients who frequently answer questions about their illness and whose responses to questions may be well rehearsed.

Table 7.10   Study design for measuring repeatability of questionnaires

- the questionnaire and the method of administration must be identical on each occasion
- at the second administration, both subject and observer must be blinded to the results of the first questionnaire
- the time to the second administration should be short enough so that the condition has not changed but long enough for the subject to have forgotten their previous reply
- the setting in which repeatability is established must be the same as the setting in which the questionnaire will be used

---

The most commonly used statistics for describing the repeatability of categorical data are kappa, the observed proportion in agreement and the average correct classification rate. Both kappa and proportion in agreement are easily calculated using most software packages.

Kappa is appropriate for assessing test-retest repeatability of self-administered questionnaires and between-observer agreement of interviewer-administered questionnaires. In essence, kappa is an estimate of the proportion in agreement between two administrations of a questionnaire after taking into account the amount of agreement that could have occurred by chance. Thus, kappa is an estimate of the difference between the observed and the expected agreement expressed as a proportion of the maximum difference and, in common with ICC, is the proportion of the variance that can be regarded as the between-subject variance.

Table 7.11 shows the format in which data need to be presented in order to calculate kappa. From this table, the observed proportion in agreement is the number of subjects who give the same reply on both occasions, that is $(61+18)/85 = 0.93$. The value for kappa, calculated using a statistics package, is 0.81.

Table 7.11	Responses on two occasions to the question 'Has your child wheezed in the last 12 months?'		
	Time 1 No	Time 1 Yes	Total
Time 2 No	61	4	65
Time 2 Yes	2	18	20
Total	63	22	85

As for correlation coefficients, a kappa value of zero represents only chance agreement and value of one represents perfect agreement. In general, a kappa above 0.5 indicates moderate agreement, above 0.7 indicates good agreement, and above 0.8 indicates very good agreement. Kappa is always a lower value than the observed proportion in agreement. However, kappa is influenced substantially by the prevalence of the positive replies, with the value increasing as the prevalence of the positive value (outcome) increases for the same proportion in agreement.

To overcome this, average correct classification rate was suggested as an alternative measurement of repeatability.[11] However, this measurement, which is usually higher than the observed proportion in agreement, has not been widely adopted. This statistic represents the probability of a consistent answer and, unlike kappa, is an 'absolute' measure of repeatability that is not influenced by prevalence. The average correct classification rate for the data shown in Table 7.11 is 0.96. In estimating the repeatability of questionnaires, we recommend that all three measurements are computed and compared in order to assess which questions provide the most reliable responses.

If there are three or more possible reply categories for a question, then a weighted kappa statistic must be calculated. In this, replies that are two or more categories from the initial response contribute more heavily to the statistic than those that are one category away from the initial response. In fact, questionnaire responses with three or more categories can be analysed using ICC, which is an approximation of weighted kappa when the number of subjects is large enough.

Repeatability and validity

The differences in study design for measuring repeatability and validity are discussed in Chapter 3. In essence, poor repeatability will always compromise the validity of an instrument because it limits accuracy, and therefore the conclusions that can be drawn from the results. However, a valid instrument may have a degree of measurement error. A problem with using ICC in isolation from other statistics to describe repeatability is that it has no dimension and is not a very responsive statistic. A high ICC may be found in the presence of a surprisingly large amount of measurement error, as indicated by the repeatability statistics computed for the data shown in Table 7.4. In isolation from other statistics, the presentation of ICC alone is usually insufficient to describe the consistency of an instrument. Because the measurement error is an absolute indication of consistency and has a simple clinical interpretation, it is a much more helpful indicator of precision.[12]

In any research study, it is important to incorporate steps to reduce measurement error and improve the validity of the study protocol. These steps may include practices such as training the observers, standardising the equipment and the calibration procedures, and blinding observers to the study group of the subjects. All of these practices will lead to the reporting of more reliable research results because they will tend to minimise both bias and measurement errors. The effects of these practices will result in a lower measurement error and a higher ICC value for the measurement tools used.

Section 2—Agreement between methods

The objectives of this section are to understand how to:
- validate different measurements or measurements using different instruments against one another;
- use various measurements to describe agreement between tests; and
- interpret graphical and statistical methods to describe agreement.

Agreement

It is important to know when measurements from the same subjects, but taken using two different instruments, can be used interchangeably. In any situation, it is unlikely that two different instruments will give identical results for all subjects. The extent to which two different methods of measuring the same variable can be compared or can be used interchangeably is called agreement between the methods. This is also sometimes called the *comparability* of the tests.

When assessing agreement, we are often measuring the criterion validity or the construct validity between two tests, which was discussed in Chapter 3. The study design for measuring agreement is exactly the same as for measuring repeatability, which is summarised in Chapter 2. The statistics that are available to estimate the agreement between two methods are shown in Table 7.12.

Table 7.12 Statistics used to measure agreement	
Both measurements continuous and units the same	Measurement error Mean-vs-differences plot Paired t-test Intra-class correlation (ICC) 95% range of agreement
Both measurements continuous and units different	Linear regression
Both measurements categorical	Kappa Sensitivity and specificity Positive and negative predictive power Likelihood ratio
One measurement categorical and one continuous	ROC curve

Continuous data and units the same

It is unlikely that two different instruments, such as two different brands of scales to measure weight, will give an identical result for all subjects. Because of this, it is important to know the extent to which the two measurements can be used interchangeably or converted from one instrument to the other and, if they are converted, how much error there is around the conversion.

If two instruments provide measurements that are expressed in the same units, then the agreement can be estimated from the measurement error or the mean within-subject difference between measurements. Because these statistics are calculated by comparing a measurement from each instrument in the same group of subjects, they are often similar to the methods described for repeatability in the previous section of this chapter. Methods of calculating measurement error can be used to estimate the bias that can be attributed to the inherent differences in the two instruments or which results from factors such as subject compliance or observer variation.

Mean-vs-differences plot

As with repeatability, important information about the extent of the agreement between two methods can be obtained by drawing up a mean-vs-difference plot.[13] Calculation of the 95 per cent range of agreement also provides important information.[14] A mean-vs-differences plot gives more information than a simple correlation plot because it shows whether there is a systematic bias in the agreement between the methods, and whether a systematic adjustment will be needed so that results from either method can be interchanged. If the slope of the regression line through the mean-vs-differences plot and the mean difference are both close to zero, no conversion factor is required. However, if the slope of the regression line through the plot is equal to zero and the mean difference is not close to zero, then the bias between the methods can be adjusted by adding or subtracting the mean difference.

The shape of the scatter in the plot conveys much information about the agreement between the measurements. As for repeatability, we recommend that the total length of the y-axis represents one-third to one-half of the length of the x-axis. If the scatter is close to the zero line, as shown for repeatability in Figure 7.3, then we can infer that there is a high level of agreement between the two instruments and that they can be used interchangeably.

Figure 7.9   Mean-vs-differences plot

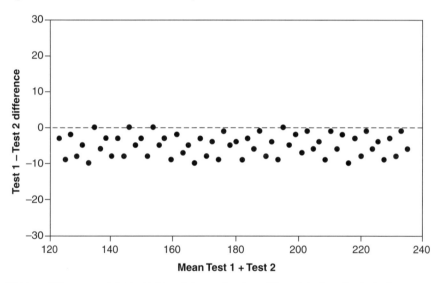

Mean-vs-differences plot of readings taken using two different test methods in the same group of subjects showing that there is good agreement with a constant difference between the measurements as indicated by a narrow scatter that is below the zero line of no difference.

A scatter that is narrow but that falls above or below the line of zero difference as shown in Figure 7.9 indicates that there is a high level of agreement between the two instruments but that a conversion factor is needed before one measurement can be substituted for the other. If the scatter is wide as shown for repeatability in Figure 7.4, then we can conclude that the two instruments do not agree well, perhaps because they are measuring different characteristics, or because one or both instruments are imprecise. An outline of a study that demonstrates this problem is shown in Example 7.2.

Figure 7.10

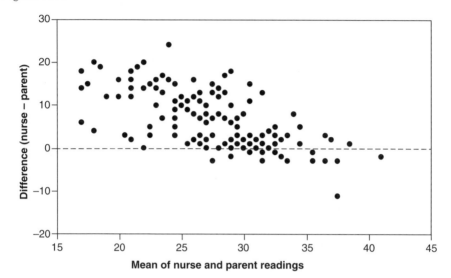

Mean of nurse and parent readings

Mean-vs-differences plot of pulse readings of infants made by the mother using fingers over the infant's wrist compared with simultaneous readings by a nursing using a stethoscope over the infant's chest.[15]

Example 7.2 Measurement of construct validity, or agreement, between two methods of measuring infants' pulse rates

Figure 7.10 shows a mean-vs-differences plot for the pulse readings of infants made by the mother using fingers over the wrist pulse of the infant compared with readings made by a nurse using a stethoscope to assess the infant's heart beat.[16] The plot shows that there is fairly poor agreement between the readings with the nurse almost always obtaining a higher reading than the parent. The shape of the plot also indicates that the construct validity at higher pulse rates is better than at lower rates. The Kendall's correlation for this plot is -0.50, $P<0.001$, which confirms the systematic bias that is evident. The ICC value is also low at 0.17, which confirms the poor agreement between the two methods. In this case, good agreement would not be expected since the nurse had the advantage of experience and the use of superior equipment designed for this purpose. In this situation, there is little point in computing the 95% range of agreement or a regression equation to convert one measurement to the other, since the parent readings are not a good estimate of the gold standard.

The presence of a consistent bias can be ascertained by computing the rank correlation coefficient for a plot. As for repeatability, a rank correlation coefficient such as Kendall's correlation coefficient, can be used to assess whether the agreement between instruments is related to the size of the measurement. A significant correlation would indicate that there is a systematic bias in the agreement between the two instruments; that is, the bias increases or decreases with the size of the measurement. This can be interpreted to mean that the difference between the measurements increases or decreases in a systematic way as the measurements become larger or smaller.

If a systematic bias exists, then the regression equation through a scatter plot of measurements taken using the two methods can be used to determine the relationship between the two measurements. The equation can then be used to convert measurements taken with one method to an approximation of the other.

The 95 per cent range of agreement

In 1986, Bland and Altman described the extent to which the methods agree as the 95 per cent range of agreement, or simply the range in which 95 per cent of the individual differences can be expected to lie.[17] This is calculated by the formula:

$$\text{95\% range} = \text{mean difference} \pm (\text{t} \times \text{SD of differences})$$

If the two measurements shown in Table 7.4 had been calculated using different types of weight scales, then:

$$\text{95\% range} = \text{mean difference} \pm (\text{t} \times \text{SD of differences})$$
$$= 0.22 + (1.96 \times 1.33)$$
$$= 0.22 \pm 2.61$$
$$= -2.39 \text{ to } 2.83 \text{ kg}$$

which indicates that we are 95 per cent certain that the measurement from the second instrument will lie within the interval of 2.39 kg less to 2.83 kg more than the measurement from the first instrument.

In a more recent publication, Bland and Altman describe the limits of agreement as the range in which 95 per cent of the difference between two measurements can be expected to lie.[18, 19] These limits are estimated around a mean difference of zero between measurements and are calculated as follows:

$$\text{95\% range} < \sqrt{2} \times 1.96 \times \text{within-subject SD}$$

in which

$$\text{within-subject SD} = \sqrt{(\text{sum of differences}^2 / 2n)}$$

If the two measurements shown in Table 7.4 had been calculated using different types of weight scales, then the 95 per cent range would be as follows:

$$95\% \text{ range} < \sqrt{2} \times 1.96 \times \text{within-subject SD}$$

$$< 1.414 \times 1.96 \times \sqrt{(\text{sum of differences}^2 / 2n)}$$

$$< 1.414 \times 1.96 \times \sqrt{(53.04 / 60)}$$

$$< 1.414 \times 1.96 \times 0.94$$

$$< 2.61 \text{ kg}$$

This can be interpreted to mean that we can be 95 per cent certain that the difference between the two weight scales being used to make the same measurement in any subject would be less than 2.61 kg. In practice, the judgment of good agreement needs to be based on clinical experience. Obviously, two instruments can only be used interchangeably if this range is not of a clinically important magnitude. In addition, the repeatability of each method has to be considered because an instrument with poor repeatability will never agree well with another instrument.

Glossary

Term	Meaning
Construct validity	Extent to which a test agrees with another test
Criterion validity	Extent to which a test agrees with the gold standard
Subject compliance	Extent to which a subject can perform a test correctly
Observer variation	Variation due to researchers administering tests in a non-standardised way

Continuous data and units different

Occasionally, it is important to measure the extent to which two entirely different instruments can be used to predict the measurements from one another. In this situation, estimates of measurement error are not useful because we expect the two measurements to be quite different. To estimate the extent to which one measurement predicts the other, linear regression is the most appropriate statistic and the correlation coefficient gives an indication of how much of the variation in one measurement is explained by the other.

An example of a study to measure criterion validity is shown in Example 7.3. This study was designed to measure the extent to which the true body weight of immobilised, supine children can be estimated by weighing their leg when hanging it in a sling. This is important for immobilised children who are undergoing urgent treatment or surgery and whose body weight is needed to accurately estimate their drug dose requirements. The study showed that hanging leg weight was able to predict total body weight more accurately than other measurements such as supine length.

Characteristic	Description
Example 7.3 Methodology study to measure criterion validity Haftel et al. Hanging leg weight—a rapid technique for estimating total body weight in pediatric resuscitation.[20]	
Aims	To assess the accuracy of two methods of estimating body weight
Type of study	Methodology study
Subjects	100 children undergoing general anesthesia in a hospital
Outcome measurements	Body weight measured using scales pre-anesthesia and estimated by supine length and hanging leg weight after induction of anesthesia
Data analyses	Supine length and hanging leg weight compared to the 'gold standard' body weight using regression analyses
Conclusions	Hanging leg weight was a more accurate predictor of body weight than supine length
Implications	In emergency and other situations when children are inert, their body weight can be estimated within 10% of their actual weight so that drug doses can be more accurately estimated
Strengths	• A large sample size was used so that the agreement between methods could be calculated with precision • Many of the conditions under which agreement has to be measured (Table 2.12) were fulfilled
Limitations	• It is not clear if observers were blinded to the information of body weight or the first of the two measurements taken • The comparison of R^2 values between subgroups may not have been appropriate because R^2 is influenced by the range of the data points

Both measurements categorical

The level of agreement between categorical measurements is often an important concept in testing the utility of diagnostic tests. The extent to which the presence or absence of a disease is predicted by a diagnostic test is an essential part of clinical practice, and is another aspect of agreement between test methods. Patients are often classified as the disease being present or absent on the basis of their signs, symptoms or other clinical features in addition to having the probability of their illness confirmed on the basis of diagnostic tests such as X-rays, biopsies, blood tests, etc. In this case, the ability of the diagnostic test to predict the patient's true disease status is measured by the sensitivity and specificity of the test. The method for calculating these diagnostic statistics is shown in Table 7.13.

Table 7.13 Calculation of diagnostic statistics			
	Disease present	Disease absent	Total
Test positive	a	b	a+b
Test negative	c	d	c+d
Total	a+c	b+d	

Notes: Sensitivity = a/(a+c)
Specificity = d/(b+d)
Positive predictive value = a/(a+b)
Negative predictive value = d/(c+d)
Likelihood ratio = Sensitivity/(1−specificity)

An example of the sensitivity and specificity of pre-discharge total serum bilirubin (TSB) levels of newborn infants in diagnosing subsequent significant hyperbilirubinemia has been reported[21] and is shown in Table 7.14.

Glossary

Term	Meaning
Sensitivity	Proportion of disease positive subjects who are correctly diagnosed by a positive test result
Specificity	Proportion of disease negative subjects who are correctly diagnosed by a negative test result
Positive predictive value	Proportion of subjects with a positive test result who have the disease
Negative predictive value	Proportion of subjects with a negative test result who do not have the disease

Table 7.14 Example of diagnostic statistics[22]			
	Hyperbilirubinemia present	Hyperbilirubinemia absent	Total
TSB test positive	114 a	414 b	528
TSB test negative	12	d 2300	2312
Total	126	2714	2840

From the data in Table 7.14, the sensitivity of the diagnostic test, that is the proportion of newborn infants who were correctly identified by the TSB test, is calculated as follows:

Sensitivity = proportion of newborn infants with hyperbilirubinemia who had a positive test

= a/a+c

= 114/126

= 0.905

The specificity of the test, that is the proportion of newborn infants who had a negative screening test and who did not have iron deficiency is calculated as follows:

Specificity = proportion of newborn infants who had a negative test but no iron deficiency

= d/b+d

= 2300/2714

= 0.847

The sensitivity and specificity of tests are useful statistics because they do not alter if the prevalence of the subjects with a positive diagnosis is different between study situations. As a result, the statistics can be applied in different clinical populations and settings. Thus, these statistics can be reliably compared between different studies especially studies that use different selection criteria, or can be used to compare the diagnostic potential of different tests.

However, the purpose of a diagnostic test is usually to enable a more accurate diagnosis in a patient who presents for treatment, that is to be inductive. For this, it is more useful to know the probability that the test will give the correct diagnosis than to know the sensitivity and specificity.[23] The predictive power of a test is judged by the positive predictive value

(PPV), which can be calculated as the proportion of patients with a positive diagnostic test result who are correctly diagnosed. In addition, the negative predictive value (NPV) is also useful—this is the proportion of patients with a negative diagnostic test result who are correctly ruled out of having the disease.

From Table 7.14, the positive and negative predictive values of the TSB test are calculated as follows:

Positive predictive value = proportion with TSB test positive have hyperbilirubinemia

$$= a/a+b$$
$$= 114/528$$
$$= 0.216$$

Negative predictive value = proportion with TSB test negative without hyperbilirubinemia

$$= d/c+d$$
$$= 2300/2312$$
$$= 0.995$$

Although essential in a clinical setting, the major limitation of positive and negative predictive values is that they are strongly influenced by the prevalence of subjects with a positive diagnosis. Both the PPV and NPV will be higher when the prevalence of the disease is common and, when a disease is rare, the positive predictive value will never be close to one. In the example above, the positive predictive value is low because only 4 per cent of babies (114/2840) have a TSB test positive and also develop hyperbilirubinemia. In this situation, we can be more sure that a negative test indicates no disease and less sure that a positive result really indicates that the disease is present.[24]

Because both the positive and negative predictive values are heavily dependent on the prevalence of the disease in the study sample, they are difficult to apply in other clinical settings or compare between different diagnostic tests. These statistics cannot be applied in clinical settings in which the profile of the patients is different from the sample for which PPV and NPV were calculated, or between studies in which the prevalence of the disease is different.

Likelihood ratio

A statistic that is inductive and that avoids these problems of comparability between studies and applicability in different clinical settings is the likelihood ratio. The likelihood ratio gives an indication of the value of a diagnostic test in increasing the certainty of a positive diagnosis. The likelihood ratio is the probability of a patient having a positive diagnostic test result if they truly have the disease compared to the corresponding probability if they were disease-free.[25] As such, the likelihood ratio indicates the value of a test in increasing the certainty of a positive diagnosis.

The likelihood ratio is calculated as follows:

$$\text{Likelihood ratio} = \text{Sensitivity}/(1 - \text{Specificity})$$

that is, the true positive rate as a proportion of the false positive rate. This can be used to convert the pre-test estimate that a patient will have the disease into a post-test estimate, thereby providing a more effective diagnostic statistic than PPV.

For the data shown in Table 7.14:

$$\text{Likelihood ratio} = 0.905/(1 - 0.847)$$
$$= 5.92$$

The following statistics can also be calculated from Table 7.14:

$$\text{Pre-test prevalence (p) of TSB positive} = (a+c)/\text{Total}$$
$$= 528/2840$$
$$= 0.186$$

$$\text{Pre-test odds of subjects having hyperbilirubinemia} = p/(1 - p)$$
$$= 0.186/(1 - 0.186)$$
$$= 0.23$$

The likelihood ratio of the diagnostic test can then be used to calculate the post-test odds of a patient having a disease as follows:

$$\text{Post-test odds} = \text{pre-test odds} \times \text{likelihood ratio}$$
$$= 0.23 \times 5.92$$
$$= 1.32$$

The higher the likelihood ratio, the more useful the test will be for diagnosing disease.[26] The increase of a newborn having hyperbilirubinemia from a pre-test odds of 0.23 to a post-test odds of 1.32 gives an indication of the value of conducting a newborn screening test of TSB when ruling in or ruling out the presence of hyperbilirubinemia. A simple nomogram for using the likelihood ratio to convert a pre-test odds to a post-test odds has been published by Sackett et al.[27]

Confidence intervals

Of course, none of the diagnostic statistics above are calculated without a degree of error because all have been estimated from a sample of subjects. To measure the certainty of the statistics, confidence intervals can be calculated as for any proportion and the level of precision will depend on the number of subjects with and without the diagnosis. For the diagnostic statistics shown in Table 7.14, the estimates shown as percentages with their 95 per cent confidence intervals calculated using the computer program CIA[28] are as follows:

> Sensitivity = 90.5% (95% CI 84.0, 95.0)
> Specificity = 84.7% (95% CI 83.4, 86.1)
> Postive predictive value = 21.6% (95% CI 18.1, 25.1)
> Negative predictive value = 99.5% (95% CI 99.1, 99.7)

The confidence intervals for specificity and negative predictive value are quite small and reflect the large number of newborn infants who had negative tests. Similarly, the larger confidence intervals around sensitivity and positive predictive value reflect the smaller number of infants with positive tests. The confidence intervals around some diagnostic statistics can be surprisingly large and reflect the imprecision always obtained when estimates are calculated from samples in which the number of subjects is relatively small.

One measurement continuous and one categorical

Sometimes it is important to know the extent to which continuously distributed measurements, such as biochemical tests, can predict the presence or absence of a disease. In this situation, a cut-off value that delineates a 'normal' from an 'abnormal' test result is usually required. The cut-off point that most accurately predicts the disease can be calculated by plotting a receiver-operating characteristic (ROC) curve.[29]

To construct a ROC curve, the sensitivity and specificity of the measurement in predicting the disease is computed, as a percentage, for several different cut-off points along the distribution of the continuous variable. Then, for each cut-off value, the sensitivity (the rate of true positives) is plotted against 1 – specificity (the rate of false positives). An example of a ROC plot is shown in Figure 7.11.

In the study shown in Table 7.14, the cut-off point for a positive TSB test was defined as a value above the 75 per cent percentile. Although other cut-off points of 40 per cent and 90 per cent were investigated, the cut-off of above the 75 per cent percentile had the highest predictive value as indicated by a ROC plot.[30]

Figure 7.11 Receiver operating curve (ROC)

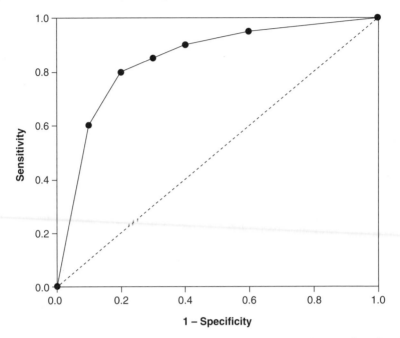

ROC curve showing the sensitivity of a test measurement plotted against 1 – Specificity for various cut-off values of the test measurement constructed from the results of Bhutani.

In practice, the larger the area under the curve then the more reliable the measurement is for distinguishing between disease and non-disease groups. A completely useless test would follow the line of identity across the plot.[31] A cut-off point that maximises the rate of true positives (sensitivity) whilst minimising the rate of false positives (1 – specificity) is obviously the point at which the test best discriminates between subjects with or without the disease of interest. This cut-off point is indicated by the point on the curve that is closest to the top of the y-axis, that is the top left-hand corner of the figure.

The ability of a test to discriminate between two different illness conditions can be assessed by plotting a ROC curve for one illness on the same graph as the other. The plot with the largest area under the curve and which passes closest to the upper left-hand corner of the figure will indicate which of the two disease conditions the test can most accurately identify.[32, 33]

Section 3—Relative risk, odds ratio and number needed to treat

The objectives of this section are to understand how to:
- describe associations between categorical exposure and outcome variables; and
- translate the association into a clinically meaningful statistic.

Measures of association

The relative risk (RR), odds ratio (OR) and number needed to treat (NNT) are statistics that are used to describe the risk of a disease or outcome in subjects who are exposed to an environmental factor, an active intervention or a treatment. The relative risk and odds ratio are sometimes described using the alternative nomenclature shown in Table 7.15.

Table 7.15 Terms used to describe relative risk and odds ratio	
Term	Alternative terms
Relative risk (RR)	Risk ratio Rate ratio Relative rate Incidence rate ratio
Odds ratio (OR)	Relative odds Cross ratio

To calculate these statistics, the data need to be summarised as a 2×2 table as shown in Table 7.16. For clinical epidemiology, the subjects in the 'exposed' group are the patients who are in the active treatment group or who have undergone a new clinical intervention, and the subjects in the 'not exposed' group are the patients in the control group.

Table 7.16	Format used to measure odds ratios, relative risk and number needed to treat		
	Exposed	Not exposed	Total
Disease present	a	b	a+b
Disease absent	c	d	c+d
Total	a+c	b+d	Total sample

Relative risk

Relative risk (RR) is usually used to describe associations between exposures and outcomes in prospective cohort or cross-sectional studies. This statistic cannot be used for data from case-control studies. Relative risk is computed by comparing the rate of illness in the exposed and unexposed groups. Relative risk is a useful statistic that can be computed from population studies in which subjects are exposed as a result of personal choice (e.g. smoking), or as a result of occupational exposures (e.g. asbestos) or environmental exposures (e.g. industrial air pollutants).

Relative risk is calculated as follows from a table in the format shown in Table 7.16:

$$RR = \frac{a/(a+c)}{b/(b+d)}$$

Table 7.17 shows the prevalence of bronchitis in early infancy measured retrospectively in 8–11 year-old children studied in a large cross-sectional population study and categorised according to exposure to parental smoking.

Table 7.17	Population study of 8–11 year-old children in which information of parental smoking and bronchitis in the child in early life were collected retrospectively[34]		
	Exposed to parental smoking	Not exposed	Total
Bronchitis in infancy	97 (29%)	87 (18%)	184 (22%)
No bronchitis in infancy	244	411	655
Total	341	498	839

From the data shown in Table 7.17, the relative risk of children having bronchitis in infancy if they are exposed to parental smoking is as follows:

$$RR = 97/341 \; / \; 87/498$$
$$= 0.284 \; / \; 0.175$$
$$= 1.62$$

This statistic is simply the proportion of subjects with infancy bronchitis in the exposed group (29 per cent) divided by the proportion in the non-exposed group (18 per cent). The 95 per cent confidence intervals around the relative risk are based on logarithms. The use of logarithms gives intervals that are asymmetric around the relative risk, that is the upper limit is wider than the lower limit when the numbers are anti-logged. This is a more accurate estimate of the confidence interval than could be obtained using other methods. Because of the complexity in the calculations, the confidence intervals are best calculated using computer software. For the above example, the relative risk and its 95 per cent confidence intervals are as follows:

$$RR = 1.62 \; (95\% \; CI \; 1.26, \; 2.10)$$

Relative risk differs from the odds ratio because it is usually time dependent; that is, influenced by the time taken for the disease to develop. Because relative risk is the ratio of two cumulative risks, it is important to take the time period into account when interpreting the risk or when comparing different estimates. In some cases, relative risk is most accurate over a short time period, although not too short because the disease has to have time to develop. Over a long time period, the value may approach unity, for example if the outcome is risk of death then over a long period all subjects in both groups will eventually die and the risk will become 1.0.

Odds ratio

The odds ratio (OR) is an estimate of risk that can be calculated in studies such as case-control studies when the relative risk cannot be estimated because the proportions of cases and controls is determined by the sampling method. Because the odds ratio only closely approximates to relative risk when the exposure is rare, the magnitude of these two statistics can be quite different, especially when the exposure rate is a common event.

The odds ratio is the odds of exposure in the group with disease (cases) compared to the odds in the non-exposed group (controls). From a table in the format shown in Table 7.16, the odds ratio is calculated as follows:

$$\text{Odds ratio} = a/c \; / \; b/d$$
$$= ad \; / \; bc$$

This statistic was developed for the analysis of case-control studies, in which the prevalence of the disease does not approximate to the prevalence in the community. However, odds ratios are now used to summarise data from cohort and cross-sectional studies following the increased availability of logistic regression, which is a multivariate analysis that is often used to calculate odds ratios that are adjusted for the effects of other confounders or risk factors.

Figure 7.12   Calculation of odds ratio

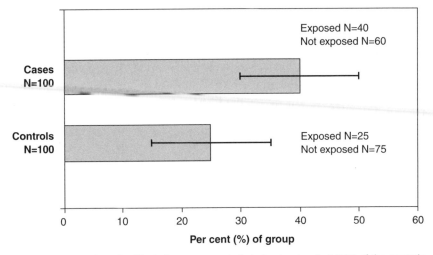

Two theoretical samples of subjects in a case-control study showing that 25% of the controls have been exposed to a factor of interest compared to 40% of the cases.

Figure 7.12 shows an example of a study in which 40 of the 100 cases were exposed to the factor of interest compared with 25 of the 100 controls. In this case, the odds ratio would be as follows:

$$OR = 40/60 \;/\; 25/75$$
$$= 2.0$$

The size of this statistic shows how the odds ratio can over-estimate the relative risk. Although the odds ratio is 2.0, the cases in this example do not have twice the rate of exposure as the controls.

From the data shown in Table 7.17, the odds ratio for children to have had a respiratory infection if they had been exposed to parental smoking is calculated as follows:

$$OR = a/c \;/\; b/d$$
$$= 97/244 \;/\; 87/411$$
$$= 1.88$$

This number can also be interpreted as the odds of children having been exposed to parental smoking if they had bronchitis in early life, which is calculated as follows:

$$OR = a/b \; / \; c/d$$
$$= 97/87 \; / \; 244/411$$
$$= 1.88$$

As with relative risk, the 95 per cent confidence intervals are best calculated using a computer program because of the complexity of the calculations. For odds ratio, an alternative method is to calculate the confidence intervals from the standard error (SE) that is produced using logistic regression. Logistic regression can be used with only one explanatory variable (in this case, parental smoking) and then produces an unadjusted estimate of the odds ratio with a standard error that is usually shown in logarithmic units.

For the example above, the calculation of the 95 per cent confidence intervals is as follows where the OR is 1.88 and the SE of 0.168 in logarithmic units has been calculated using logistic regression:

$$95\% \; CI = exp \; (log_e \; OR \; \pm \; (SE \times 1.96))$$
$$= exp \; (log_e \; (1.88) \; \pm \; (0.168 \times 1.96))$$
$$= 1.35, \; 2.62$$

Adjusted odds ratios

When confounding occurs, it is important to remove the effect of the confounder from the odds ratio that describes the association between an exposure and an outcome. For example, in Figure 7.13, factor A is a confounder in the relation between factor B and the disease outcome. Thus, the effects of factor A, as shown by the higher prevalence of disease in group 2 compared to group 1, have to be removed from group 3 before the true association between exposure B and the disease can be computed. This process can be undertaken using logistic regression.

Odds ratios calculated this way are called adjusted odds ratios and are less dependent on the effects of known confounders. This method of adjusting for the effects of confounder is the weakest method possible, but does not need as large a sample size as other methods such as matching or stratification (see Chapter 3).

Health science research

Figure 7.13   Separating multiple effects

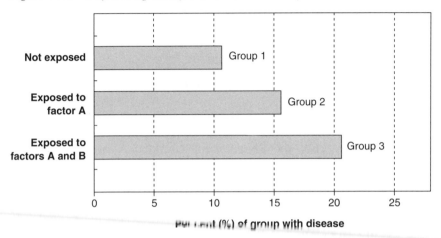

Three theoretical groups of subjects showing that 12% of the non-exposed group 1 have a disease, compared to 16% of group 2 who have been exposed to factor A and 22% of group 3 who have been exposed to both factor A and factor B.

Interpretation of confidence intervals

When interpreting the significance of either an odds ratio or relative risk, it is important to consider both the size of the effect and the precision of the estimate. If the 95 per cent confidence interval around an odds ratio or a relative risk encompasses the value of 1.0 then the effect is not statistically significant. However, we also need to examine the upper confidence interval to make a judgment about whether it falls in a clinically important range. It is important to judge whether to accept a true negative conclusion or whether to conclude that a type II error may have occurred, that is the odds ratio indicates a clinically important risk but has failed to reach statistical significance because the sample size is too small. This can be a problem in studies in which the sample size is small and logistic regression is used to test the effects of several factors simultaneously.

Figure 7.14 shows an example in which we can be certain of a true positive effect of factor A, or a true protective effect of factor D. The effect measured for factor B is larger than that for factor A but the estimate is less precise, as indicated by the wide confidence intervals. In some cases, such as for factor C, the effect may be ambiguous because it is clinically important in magnitude but has wide 95 per cent confidence intervals that overlap the value of unity. Thus, we cannot be 95 per cent certain whether factor C has a protective or risk effect on the outcome.

Figure 7.14   Odds ratios

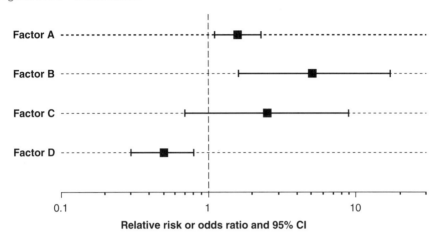

Relative risk or odds ratio and 95% CI

Four odds ratios demonstrating the importance of taking both the size and direction of the odds ratio together with its precision as indicated by the 95% confidence intervals into account when interpreting the results of a study.

Comparison of odds ratio and relative risk

Both the relative risk and the odds ratio can be difficult to interpret. In some cases, the absolute effect of the exposure in the two study groups may differ and the relative risk and odds ratio may be the same, or the absolute effect may be the same and the relative risk and odds ratio may be different. For example, if we halve the prevalence of the outcome (bronchitis in infancy) shown in Table 7.17 from 22 per cent to 11 per cent in both the exposed and the non-exposed groups then the numbers will be as shown in Table 7.18.

Table 7.18   Data from Table 7.17 modified to reduce prevalence of infancy bronchitis in both the exposed and non-exposed groups to half the prevalence measured in the actual study

	Exposed to parental smoking	Not exposed	Total
Bronchitis in infancy	48 (14%)	44 (9%)	92 (11%)
No bronchitis in infancy	293	454	747
Total	341	498	839

From Table 7.18, the relative risk will 1.59 and the odds ratio will be 1.69, which are very close to the estimates of 1.62 and 1.88 respectively that were calculated from the data shown in Table 7.17. However, if the prevalence in the non-exposed group only is halved, then the numbers will be as shown in Table 7.19.

Table 7.19	Data from Table 7.17 modified to reduce prevalence of infancy bronchitis in the non-exposed group only to half that measured in the actual study		
	Exposed to parental smoking	Not exposed	Total
Bronchitis in infancy	97 (29%)	44 (9%)	184
No bronchitis in infancy	244	454	655
Total	341	498	839

From the data in Table 7.19, the relative risk is 3.21 and the odds ratio is 4.10, which is very different from the estimates calculated from Tables 7.17 and 7.18. Thus, a large difference in estimates occurs if the prevalence of the outcome changes in only one of the exposure groups, but similar estimates of effect can occur when the prevalence changes with a similar magnitude in both groups.

Both the odds ratio and the relative risk have advantages and disadvantages when used in some situations. The features of both of these statistics are shown in Table 7.20.

Table 7.20	Features of odds ratio and relative risk estimates
Odds ratio	Relative risk
• results can be combined across strata using Mantel-Haenszel methods	• results are difficult to combine across strata
• can be used to summarise data from most studies	• can only be used for data from studies with a randomly selected sample, e.g. cohort and cross-sectional studies
• give an estimate of risk when the prevalence of the outcome is not known	• can be used to calculate attributable risk

Although the odds ratio and relative risk always go in the same direction, discrepancies between them can be large enough to become misleading. For this reason, it is better to limit the use of odds ratios to case-control studies and logistic regression analyses.[35] For the same data set, the odds ratio will be larger than the relative risk and thus may overestimate the 'true' association between the disease and exposure under investigation, especially for diseases that are a common event. Because of this, the odds ratio has been criticised as a statistic with which to report the results of randomised controlled trials in which an accurate estimate of effect is required.[36] However, for the data shown in Table 7.17, the odds ratio is 1.88 and the relative risk is very close at 1.62.

The odds ratio only gives a good approximation to the relative risk when treatment or exposure rate is a relatively rare event and the sample size is large and balanced between the exposed and non-exposed group. In cohort and cross-sectional studies, the odds ratio and relative risk can be quite different, especially when the exposure rate is a common event.

Table 7.21 Results of an intervention study to test the effects of a smoking prevention program

	Exposed to intervention	Not exposed	Total
Smoker	20 (20%)	40 (40%)	60 (30%)
Non-smoker	80	60	140
Total	100	100	200

In practice, the difference between the odds ratio and the relative risk becomes smaller as the prevalence of the disease outcome decreases. For odds ratios over 2.5 that are calculated from cohort or cross-sectional studies, a correction of the odds ratio may be required to obtain a more accurate estimate of association.[37] For example, from the data shown in Table 7.21, the odds ratio is 2.6 and the relative risk is 2.0. However, Table 7.22 shows that these two statistics become increasingly closer as the prevalence of smokers decreases.

Table 7.22 Comparison between relative risk and odds ratio when the prevalence of the outcome changes

% smokers in intervention	% smokers in control group	Odds ratio	Relative risk
20	40	2.60	2.0
10	20	2.25	2.0
5	10	2.10	2.0
1	2	2.02	2.0

Number needed to treat

The odds ratio is not a useful statistic at the patient level because it is difficult to apply to an individual. However, a statistic called the number needed to treat (NNT) can be calculated from the results of studies such as randomised controlled trials and is useful in clinical practice.[38] This number can also be calculated from meta-analyses, which combine the results from several trials. The number needed to treat is an estimate of the number of patients who need to receive a new treatment for one additional patient to benefit. Clearly, a treatment that saves one life for every ten patients treated is better than a treatment that saves one life for every 50 patients treated.[39]

Table 7.23	Results from a randomised controlled trial to test the efficacy of a new treatment to prevent death as presented by Guyatt et al.[40]		
	Treatment	Controls	Total
Died	15 (15%)	20 (20%)	35 (17.5%)
Survived	85	80	165
Total	100	100	200

To estimate NNT[41] from Table 7.23, the absolute risk reduction (ARR); that is, the difference in the proportion of events between the two treatment groups, needs to be calculated as follows:

$$\text{Absolute risk reduction} = 20\% - 15\%$$
$$= 5\%, \text{ or } 0.05$$

The number needed to treat is then calculated as the reciprocal of this risk reduction as follows:

$$\text{NNT} = 1/\text{ARR}$$
$$= 1/0.05$$
$$= 20$$

This indicates that twenty patients will need to receive the new treatment to prevent one death. This effect has to be balanced against the cost of the treatment, the risk of death if the patient is not treated and the risk of any adverse outcomes if the patient is treated. Obviously, when there is no risk reduction, ARR will be zero and NNT then becomes infinity.

However, when NNT becomes negative it gives an indication of the number of patients that need to be treated to cause harm.

The 95 per cent confidence interval (CI) for ARR is calculated as for any difference in proportions.[42] These intervals are then inverted and exchanged to produce the 95 per cent CIs for NNT.[43] In the example above:

$$95\% \text{ CI for ARR} = -0.16, 0.06$$

and therefore,

$$\text{NNT} = 20 \ (95\% \text{ CI} - 18.2 \text{ to } 6.5)$$

This is interpreted as NNT = 20 (95% CI NN to benefit=6.5 to infinity to NN to harm=18.2).[44] A method for plotting NNT with its 95 per cent confidence intervals on an axis that encompasses infinity as the central value has been described by Altman.[45]

It is important to recognise that there is no association between the P value, which is an estimate of whether the difference between the treatment groups is due to chance, and the NNT, which is the clinical impact of a treatment.[46] It is also important to remember that, when applying NNT in clinical decision-making, the clinical population must be similar to the study population from which NNT was derived.

Section 4—Matched and paired analyses

The objectives of this section are to understand how to:
- conduct matched or non-matched analyses;
- decide whether matched case-control studies are reported correctly; and
- control for confounders in case-control studies.

Matched and paired studies

In case-control studies, cases are often matched with controls on the basis of important confounders. This study design can be more effective in removing the effects of confounders than designs in which confounding factors are measured and taken into account at a later stage in the analyses. However, the correct matched statistical analyses must be used in all studies in which matching is used in the study design or in the recruitment process.

The strengths and limitations of matched case-control studies were discussed in Chapter 2. The appropriate analyses for this type of study are methods designed for paired data, including the use of conditional logistic regression. In effect, the sample size in matched studies is the number of pairs of cases and controls and not the total number of subjects. This effective sample size also applies to all studies in which paired data are collected, such as studies of twins, infection rates in kidneys, or changes in events over time. The effect of pairing has a profound influence on both the statistical power of the study and the precision of any estimates of association, such as the 95 per cent confidence intervals around an odds ratio.

The basic concepts of using analyses that take account of matching and pairing are shown in Table 7.24.

Table 7.24   Concepts of matched and paired analyses

- if matching or pairing is used in the design, then matched or paired statistics must be used in the data analyses
- the outcomes and exposures of interest are the differences between each case and its matched control or between pairs, that is the within-pair variation
- the between-subject variation is not of interest and may obscure the true result
- treating the cases and controls as independent samples, or the paired measurements as independent data, will artificially inflate the sample size and lead to biased or inaccurate results

---

Presentation of non-matched and matched ordinal data

In studies such as cross-sectional and case-control studies, the number of units in the analyses is the total number of subjects. However, in matched and paired analyses, the number of units is the number of matches or pairs. An example of how the odds ratio and difference in proportions is calculated in non-matched and matched analyses is shown in Tables 7.25 and 7.26. Confidence intervals, which are best obtained using a statistics package program, can be calculated around both the odds ratios and the differences in proportions.

Table 7.25   Calculation of chi-square and odds ratio for non-matched or non-paired data

	Exposure positive	Exposure negative	
Cases	a	b	a+b
Controls	c	d	c+d
Total	a+c	b+d	N

Notes: Continuity-adjusted chi-square $= \dfrac{N\,(|ad - bc| - N/2)^2}{(a+b)(c+d)(a+c)(b+d)}$

Odds ratio $= (a/c)/(b/d)$

Difference in proportions $= (a/(a+c)) - (b/(b+d))$

Table 7.26	Calculation of chi-square and odds ratio for matched or paired data		
	Exposure positive	Exposure negative	
Cases	a	b	a+b
Controls	c	d	c+d
Total	a+c	b+d	N

Notes: McNemar's chi-square $= \dfrac{(|b-c| - 1)^2}{(b+c)}$

Matched odds ratio $= b/c$

Difference in proportions $= (b-c)/N$

The difference in the statistics obtained using these two methods is shown in Table 7.27. In this example, the data were matched in the study design stage and therefore the matched analyses are the correct statistics with which to present the results.

In the upper table in Table 7.27, the effective sample size is the total number of children in the study whereas in the lower table, the effective size of the sample is the number of pairs of children. The unmatched odds ratio of 3.0 under-estimates the risk of children having infection if they are exposed to maternal smoking which is 4.8 when calculated from the matched data. Also, although the difference in proportions is the same in both calculations and indicates that the rate of infection is 27 per cent higher in exposed children, the matched analysis provides a less biased estimate with more precise confidence intervals.

The odds ratio will usually be quite different for the same data set when matched and unmatched analyses are used. If the subjects have been matched in the study design, then the matched odds ratio and its confidence interval will provide a more precise estimate of effect than the unmatched odds ratio. If non-matched and matched analyses give the same estimate of the odds ratio, this suggests that the matching characteristics were not confounders. Even if the effects are the same, confidence intervals using a matched approach should be used because they are more accurate.

Using more than one control for each case

To increase statistical power, more than one control can be recruited for each case. In this situation, the differences between the cases and controls are still the outcomes of interest but the effective sample size is the number

Table 7.27 Calculating non-matched and matched statistics in a case-control study in which 86 children with respiratory infection were age and gender matched with 86 children who had not had a respiratory infection and exposure to maternal smoking was measured

i. Non-matched presentation and statistics

	Exposed	Not exposed	Total
Infection (cases)	56 (65.1%)	30 (34.9%)	86 (100%)
No infection (controls)	33 (38.4%)	53 (61.6%)	86 (100%)
Total	89	83	172

Notes: Continuity-adjusted chi-square = 11.27, $P<0.0005$

Odds ratio = 3.0 (95% CI 1.6, 5.5)

Difference in proportions = 26.7% (95% CI 12.4, 41.1)

ii. Matched presentation and statistics

	Control exposed	Control not exposed	
Case exposed	27 (31.4%)	29 (33.7%)	56
Case not exposed	6 (7.0%)	24 (27.9%)	30
Total	33	53	86
			100%

Notes: McNemar's chi-square = 13.82, $P<0.0004$

Matched odds ratio = 4.8 (95% CI 2.0, 11.6)

Difference in proportions = 26.7% (95% CI 13.3, 35.4)

of control subjects. Thus, if 50 cases and 100 controls are enrolled, the number of matched pairs would be 100. Because there are 100 matches, the data from each case is used twice and the data from each control is used once only. This method can also be used if data for some controls are missing because a match could not be found. If 40 cases had two matched controls and 10 cases had only one matched control, the sample size would then be 90 pairs. The bias that results from using the data for some cases in more than one pair is not so large as the bias that would result from treating the data as unpaired samples.

Logistic regression

Adjusted odds ratios are calculated for non-matched data using logistic regression, and can be calculated for matched data using conditional logistic regression. Conditional logistic regression is particularly useful in studies in which there is more than one control for each case subject, including studies in which the number of control subjects per case is not consistent.

Obviously, in the results shown in Table 7.27, the effects of age and gender on rate of infection cannot be investigated since they were the matching variables. However, interactions between another exposure factor, say breastfeeding, and age could be investigated by including the interaction factor age*breastfeeding without including the main effect of age. Clearly, length of time of breastfeeding will be closely related to the age of the infant and because the subjects are matched on age, the effect of breastfeeding may be under-estimated if included in the model.

Presentation of matched and paired continuous data

As with ordinal data, the outcome of interest when estimating differences in continuous variables in matched or paired studies is the difference in the outcome variable between each of the pairs. Thus, the sample size is also the number of pairs of subjects. A statistical difference in outcomes for the cases and controls can be tested using a paired t-test. Alternatively, multiple regression can be used with the outcome variable being the difference in outcomes between each pair and the explanatory variables being the differences in the explanatory variable between the pairs, or between each case and control subject.

Section 5—Exact methods

Applications of exact methods

It is essential to use accurate statistical methods in any research study so that the results can be correctly interpreted. Exact statistical methods need to be used whenever the prevalence of the disease or the exposure variable in the study sample is rare. This can occur in epidemiological studies conducted by surveillance units such as the British and the Australian Paediatric Surveillance Units in which national data of the incidence and characteristics of rare diseases of childhood are collected.[47, 48] Exact methods also need to be used in clinical studies in which a small sample size can lead to very small numbers in some groups when the data are stratified. Because these situations do not conform to the assumptions required to use 'normal' statistics, specialised statistics that are called 'exact methods' are needed.

In situations where the assumptions for normal methods are not met, 'exact' methods conserve accuracy. These 'gold standard' methods give a more precise result no matter what the distribution or frequency of the data. Of course, if the assumptions for normal methods are met, then both methods give similar answers. Whenever there is any doubt about the applicability of normal statistics, the use of exact statistics will lead to a more accurate interpretation of results.

Health science research

Difference between normal and exact methods

The statistical methods that are usually used for reporting data are 'asymptotic' or 'normal' methods. These methods are based on assumptions that the sample size is large, the data are normally distributed and the condition of interest occurs reasonably frequently, say in more than 5 per cent of the population or study sample. If these assumptions are not met, as is often the case in studies of rare diseases, normal methods become unreliable and estimates of statistical significance may be inaccurate. This is especially problematic when calculating confidence intervals, or when judging the meaning of a P value that is on the margins of significance, say 0.055, and it is important to know whether the true P value is 0.03 or 0.08.

Exact methods do not rely on any assumptions about sample size or distribution. Although these methods were developed in the 1930s, they have been largely avoided because they are based on complex formulae that are not usually available in statistics packages or because they require factorial calculations that desktop computers have not been able to handle. However, technological developments in the last decade have meant that software to calculate exact methods is now more readily accessible so that the calculation of accurate statistics is no longer a problem.[49]

Incidence and prevalence statistics

The rate of occurrence of a rare disease is usually expressed as the incidence; that is, the number of new cases that occur in a defined group with a defined time period. For reporting purposes, very low incidence rates are best expressed as the number of cases of the disease per 10 000 or per 100 000 children. Examples of the denominators that are commonly used in such calculations are the number of live births, the number of children less than five years old or the number of children living in a region in a particular year. For example, an incidence rate may be reported as 10 cases/100 000 live births/year.

The term *incidence* has a very different meaning to *prevalence*. Incidence is the rate of occurrence of new cases each year whereas prevalence is calculated from the total number of cases of a given disease in a population in a specified time, for example 20 per cent of the population in the last year. The number of remissions and deaths that occur influences the prevalence rate, but has no influence on the incidence rate.

Data from the Australian Paediatric Surveillance Unit shows that, in 1994, 139 cases of Kawasaki disease were confirmed in children under fifteen years of age.[50] This was correctly reported as a incidence rate of 3.70 cases per 100 000 children less than five years of age and 0.59 cases per 100 000 children age five to fifteen years. In oral presentations and in more informal documents in which an approximation is acceptable, these rates can be expressed as being approximately one case per 27 000 children less than five years of age or one case per 17 000 children age five to fifteen years.

Glossary

Term	Explanation
Gold standard	The best method available
'Exact' methods	Accurate statistical methods that are not based on approximations
'Normal' methods	Methods based on the assumption that the data are normally distributed, the sample size is large and the outcome of interest occurs frequently
95% confidence intervals	Range in which we are 95% certain that the true population value lies

Confidence intervals

Figures of percentages, such as incidence and prevalence rates, sensitivity, specificity etc., should always be quoted with 95 per cent confidence intervals. Between the range of 10–90 per cent, confidence intervals calculated using exact and normal methods are quite similar. However, when the percentage is below 10 per cent or above 90 per cent, and especially if the sample size is quite small, then exact methods are required for calculating the 95 per cent confidence intervals. Differences between the two methods arise because normal confidence intervals are based on a normal approximation to the binomial distribution whereas exact confidence intervals are based on the Poisson distribution.

Figure 7.15 shows a series of prevalence rates estimated in a sample size of 200 subjects and calculated using exact confidence intervals. The exact confidence intervals are uneven but are accurate. In Figure 7.16, the confidence intervals have been estimated using normal methods showing how the normal estimates become increasingly inaccurate as the prevalence rate becomes lower. The confidence intervals are even around the estimate but their inaccuracy means that the lower interval extends below zero at low prevalence rates, which is a nonsense rate. Because confidence intervals are calculated in units of a percentage, they cannot exceed 100 per cent or fall below 0 per cent.

Health science research

Figure 7.15 Exact confidence intervals

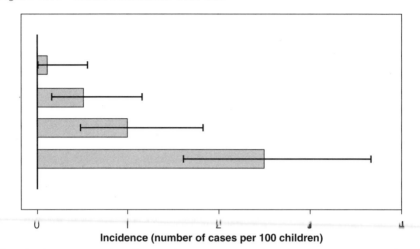

Incidence (number of cases per 100 children)

Four incidence rates of a disease that occur rarely plotted with exact 95% confidence intervals.

Figure 7.16 Normal confidence intervals

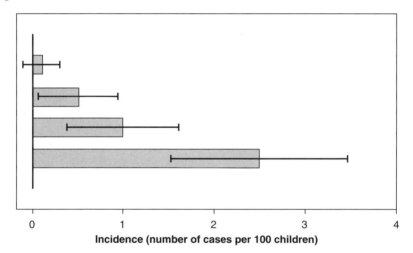

Incidence (number of cases per 100 children)

Four incidence rates of a disease that occur rarely plotted with normal 95% confidence intervals showing how nonsense values below 0% can occur when the correct statistic is not used.

Table 7.28 shows the incidence of deaths from external causes in 1995 in Australian children less than one year old, categorised according to State.[51] Confidence intervals can be calculated in this type of study even when no cases are found; that is, when the incidence rate is zero. In most studies in which only a sample of the population is enrolled, the 95 per cent confidence intervals are used to convey an estimate of the sampling error. However, 95 per cent confidence intervals can also be used when the sample is the total population and we want to make inferences about precision or compare rates, such as between States or between one year and the next, whilst taking the size of the population into account.

Table 7.28 Number and incidence (cases per 10 000 children) of deaths due to external causes in children less than one year old in 1995

State	Number of cases	Total births	Incidence	95% CI
New South Wales	14	85 966	1.63	0.89, 2.73
Victoria	7	61 529	1.14	0.46, 2.34
Queensland	12	47 613	2.52	1.30, 4.40
South Australia	3	19 114	1.57	0.32, 4.59
Western Australia	7	24 800	2.82	1.14, 5.81
Northern Territory	0	3 535	0	0.0, 10.43
Tasmania	0	6 431	0	0.0, 5.73
Australian Capital Territory	0	4 846	0	0.0, 7.61
TOTAL	43	253 834	1.69	1.23, 2.28

From this table, we might have assumed that there was a statistically significant difference in incidence between States because there were fourteen cases in New South Wales and twelve in Queensland compared to no cases in Tasmania, the Northern Territory and the Australian Capital Territory. When these numbers are standardised for population size, the incidence rate varies from zero to 2.82 cases/100 000 children less than one year old. Whenever zero values occur in cells, as in this table, Fisher's exact test has to be used to test for between-State differences. For this table, an exact test gives a P value of $P=0.317$ which indicates that there is no significant differences between States. By plotting the data as shown in Figure 7.17, we can easily see that the 95 per cent confidence intervals for the States overlap one another to a large extent and this confirms that there is no significant difference in the incidence rates.

263

Figure 7.17   Exact confidence intervals

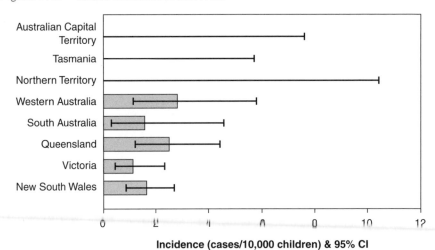

Incidence (cases/10,000 children) & 95% CI

Incidence and exact 95% confidence intervals of rate of deaths due to external causes in children less than one year of age in Australia in 1994.[52]

Glossary

Term	Explanation
Contingency table	Cross-classification of data into a table of rows and columns to indicate numbers of subjects in subgroups
Pearson's chi-square	Chi-square statistic based on assumption that the sample size is large (greater than 1000) and that there are more than 5 subjects in each cell
Continuity adjusted chi-square	Chi-square statistic adjusted for a small sample size, say of less than 1000 subjects
Fisher's exact test	Chi-square statistic used when there are less than 5 expected cases in one or more cells

Chi-square tests

We often want to test whether there is an association between a disease and other potentially explanatory factors, such as age or gender. In such cases, the data can be cross-tabulated as counts in a contingency table as shown in Table 7.29 (Personal communication, APSU). For these types of tables, a chi-square statistic that indicates whether there is a significant difference in incidence between subgroups is the correct test to use. In ordinary circumstances, Pearson's chi-square is used when the sample size is very large, that is in the thousands, or a more conservative 'continuity-corrected' chi-square test is used when the sample size is smaller, say in the hundreds. For small samples, the continuity-corrected chi-square produces a more conservative and therefore less significant value than Pearson's chi-square.

Table 7.29 Incidence of cases of Kawasaki disease in Australia in 1994 stratified by gender of the child

Gender	Non-Kawasaki cases	Cases	Total population	Incidence and 95% CI
Males	1 979 444	81	1 979 525	4.09 (3.25, 5.08)
Females	1 880 464	48	1 880 512	2.55 (1.88, 3.38)
TOTAL	3 859 908	129	3 860 037	

However, when the number of cases is very small compared to the size of the study sample, Fisher's exact test must be used. For tables larger than 2×2, exact methods must be used when more than 20 per cent of the cells have an expected count less than five. Most computer packages do not calculate exact methods for larger tables so that a specialised program is required. However, for 2×2 tables, most computer programs print out a warning and automatically calculate Fisher's exact test when there is an expected count of less than five in any cell of a contingency table. The expected cell count for any table is calculated as follows:

Expected count = (Row total × Column total)/Grand total

In Table 7.30, data about the incidence of Kawasaki disease collected by the Australian Paediatric Surveillance Unit is stratified by gender in a 2×2 table. Data from a total of 139 children were collected of whom 129 had information of gender available. From the table, the expected number of cases of Kawasaki disease for females is (1 880 512 × 129)/3 860 037 which is 62.8. Because this is quite large, Fisher's exact test is not required. The Pearson's chi-square statistic is 6.84 with P=0.01, which indicates that the incidence of disease is significantly higher in male children.

Chi-square tests are also used to investigate subsets of the data. Table 7.30 shows the data for children with Kawasaki disease categorised according to both age of diagnosis and whether the child was admitted to hospital. The expected number of children aged five years or older who

Table 7.30	Cases of Kawasaki disease in 1994 categorised according to age and admission to hospital[53]		
	Admitted to hospital	Not admitted	TOTAL
Children <5 years old	92 (91.1%)	9 (8.9%)	101
Children ≥5 years old	27 (79.4%)	7 (20.6%)	34
TOTAL	119	16	135

Note: The cells show the number of cases with the row percentage shown in brackets.

did not require admission is $(16 \times 34)/135$ which is 4.0, indicating that Fisher's exact test is required. The P value for this test is 0.12 indicating that the difference of 91 per cent children younger than five years being admitted to hospital compared to 79 per cent of older children is not statistically significant. A Pearson's chi-square value calculated for this table gives a value of 0.07, which suggests a difference of marginal significance, and outlines the importance of computing the correct statistic so that correct inferences from small P values such as this are made.

8

APPRAISING RESEARCH
PROTOCOLS

Section 1—Designing a study protocol

The objectives of this section are to provide resources for:
- designing a research study; and
- reviewing a study protocol.

Designing a research study

The studies that are most likely to provide meaningful and useful information about health care are the studies in which the most appropriate design for the setting and the most appropriate methods to answer an important research question are used. The most elegant studies are those that use the most robust study design, that use the most reliable methods to collect data and that incorporate strategies to overcome problems of bias and confounding. In addition, to attract funding, research studies must be entirely feasible to conduct, have adequate power to test the hypotheses, use appropriate statistical methods, and ensure that the conclusions that will be drawn are justified by the data.

The steps for developing a new study are shown in Table 8.1. The strengths and merits of various study designs were discussed in Chapter 2.

Table 8.1   Checklist for developing a new study
❑ Focus on the areas of health care for which the current evidence is inadequate
❑ Develop research questions into clear testable hypotheses or study aims
❑ Choose an optimal study design for each hypothesis or aim
❑ Select valid and repeatable methods to measure the outcome and exposure variables
❑ Identify and minimise potential effects of bias and confounding
❑ Plan the statistical methods needed to test each hypothesis
❑ Prepare study protocol and timelines
❑ Obtain ethical approval
❑ Estimate budget
❑ Identify appropriate funding bodies and apply for funding

It is vital to ensure that a study protocol is complete in that it explains the purpose of the study and addresses all of the fundamental design issues. Study protocols that adhere to these standards will be regarded more highly by the scientific community, including peer reviewers and the scientific advisory, ethics and granting committees.

The checklists that follow in this chapter are intended as reminders of problems that need to be addressed in order to design the best possible research study for the question or questions being asked. These checklists can also be used when reviewing protocols prepared by other researchers to ensure that no fundamental flaws in study design have been overlooked. Other checklists that have been developed to minimise the effects of bias have been published in the literature.[1]

Glossary

Term	Meaning
Null hypothesis	A hypothesis stating that there is no significant difference or relationship between two variables
A priori or alternate hypothesis	A hypothesis that states the direction of the relationship between two variables
Topic sentence	A sentence used at the beginning of a paragraph which summarises the topic of the paragraph
Research ethics	Procedures in place to ensure that the welfare of the subject is placed above the needs of the research investigator

Core checklist

A core checklist that applies to all studies is shown in Table 8.2. This checklist is intended for use in combination with the supplementary checklists shown in Tables 8.3 to 8.5 that have been specifically designed for methodology studies, clinical trials and epidemiological studies respectively. Each checklist shows the issues that need to be addressed in order to develop a well thought out protocol with a rigorous scientific design.

Most studies are planned with the ultimate intention of collecting information that can be used to improve health care. It is important to think carefully about how new results from a research study be used and particularly about whether the study is intended to improve knowledge, medical care, clinical understanding or public health.

Aims and hypotheses

The aims or hypotheses that arise from the research question need to be specific, succinct and testable. As such, each hypothesis should be encapsulated in a single short sentence. Remember that hypotheses that are non-specific, complex or have multiple clauses usually reflect a lack of clarity in thinking and make it difficult for reveiwers and granting panels to discern the exact aims of the study.

This first section must be written clearly because it sets the scene for the rest of the document. It is preferable to have only two or three clear specific hypotheses or specific aims—having too many often confuses rather than clarifies the main issues. It is usually more practical and clearer for the reviewer if hypotheses are presented for experimental study designs and aims are presented for descriptive studies and, for clarity, to avoid having both.

The decision of whether to state the hypothesis as a null hypothesis is a personal one—it is often more straightforward to simply have an a priori hypothesis. It is helpful if the aims or hypotheses are numbered in order of importance so that they can be referred to in later stages in the protocol.

The aims and hypotheses section should also have a paragraph that states very clearly what the study will achieve and why. Many researchers find it easy to succinctly verbalise why they want to conduct their study, but have difficulty writing it down. It is therefore a useful exercise to imagine what you would say to a friend or a family member if they asked why you were doing the study and then, once you had told them, they replied 'so what?'. If the aims and importance of the study can be conveyed in simple, plain language to people to whom research is a mystery, then they will also be easily understood by other scientists whose role is to peer review the protocol.

Background

The background section is like the introduction of a journal article—it needs to describe what is known and what is not known, and to justify why this study is needed. To make this section more readable, liberal sub-headings can be used together with short paragraphs that begin with topic sentences. This section can be used to 'sell' the project by including information about prior experience in the field, any pilot data, the relationship of this project to previous studies, and reasons why this study will provide new and exciting information.

Research methods

The methods section is the part of the protocol that needs most time to think through—this section should be flawless, and should be linked directly to the specific aims or hypotheses. In making this section clear, tables, figures and time-lines are essential for clarifying the research process that will be used.

This section must be comprehensive. All of the details of the study design should be outlined, together with the subject characteristics and recruitment procedures, the approximate size of the pool of subjects available, the sample size, and the treatment or intervention details. This will allow reviewers to judge how generalisable the study results will be and how the effects of bias and confounders will be minimised. Remember to include details of how any potential problems that could be anticipated will be dealt with, and to address any issues of feasibility.

Statistical methods

The statistical methods section must outline how the data being collected will be used to test each of the study hypotheses or fulfil each aim. This section should include a description of the type of data that will be collected, for example whether it will be continuous, normally distributed, or categorical.

For each aim or hypothesis, it is a good exercise to list all of the variables under subheadings of outcomes, alternate outcomes or surrogate variables, confounders and explanatory variables. This simplifies the process of deciding how these variables will be used in the analyses, which statistical methods will be appropriate, and which subjects will be included in or excluded from each analysis.

Remember that it is unethical to collect any data that is not needed. This can be avoided by giving details of how all of the data will ultimately be used. Finally, give details of how the results of the statistical analyses will be interpreted so that the study aims are fulfilled.

Table 8.2   Core checklist for designing or reviewing a research study

Aims—describe concisely:
- ❑ each study hypotheses and how you intend to test it
- ❑ why the study is important
- ❑ the specific hypotheses and/or aims

Significance—say how the study will lead to:
- ❑ better patient care
- ❑ better methods for research
- ❑ improved treatment or public health
- ❑ disease prevention

Background—describe:
- ❑ what is known and not known about the research topic
- ❑ why this study is needed
- ❑ your experience in the field
- ❑ the relationship of this study to existing projects
- ❑ how this study will provide new information

Study design—give concise details of:
- ❑ the study design
- ❑ the sampling methods
- ❑ the recruitment strategies
- ❑ inclusion and exclusion criteria
- ❑ sample size calculations

Bias and confounding—outline in detail:
- ❑ the representativeness of the sample
- ❑ the expected response rate
- ❑ any planned interim analyses or stopping rules
- ❑ methods to control for confounders

Conducting the study—describe:
- ❑ details of the data collection methods
- ❑ composition of the management and monitoring committees
- ❑ the location, content and documentation of the data files
- ❑ the statistical analyses that will be used
- ❑ how the results will be reported and interpreted

Budget and staff requirements—give details of:
- ❑ itemised unit costs
- ❑ justification of requests
- ❑ duties of required staff
- ❑ required staff training and/or qualifications

Methodological studies

Methodological studies are used to establish the repeatability and/or the validity of new or existing questionnaires, instruments or pieces of medical equipment that have been designed to measure outcome, confounding or exposure variables. The design and interpretation of these types of studies was discussed in Chapters 3 and 7.

There is sometimes an implicit assumption that established research methods are reliable, perhaps because they have been used for a long time or perhaps because they are the most practical method available. However, this is not always the case. Indeed, the majority of methods used in medical research have some degree of error or may lack validity. Some commonly used methods also have a surprisingly low repeatability for estimating health conditions or environmental exposures. Until rigorous studies to test the repeatability, validity and responsiveness of methods are undertaken, then the effects of the methods themselves on the interpretation of the results will not be clear.

It is essential that repeatability and validation studies are conducted whenever a new method is being introduced or whenever an existing method is being used in a study sample in which its reliability or validity is not known. There is no study design that can overcome bias that is an inevitable outcome of unreliable or imprecise instruments. Furthermore, there are no statistical methods for adjusting for the effects of unreliable or imprecise measurements at the data analyses stage of any study. For these reasons, methodology studies need to be conducted in the most rigorous way so that accurate information of the precision of research instruments is available. This will not only lead to high quality research data but also avoids the use of unnecessarily large sample sizes.

A checklist to help ensure that these issues are all addressed, and which is intended for use as a supplement to the core checklist (Table 8.2), is shown in Table 8.3.

Table 8.3   Checklist for designing or reviewing a methodology study

Study objectives—state whether the following will be measured:
- ❑ validity (face, content, construct, etc.)
- ❑ sensitivity and specificity
- ❑ repeatability of a single measurement
- ❑ agreement between instruments or between observers
- ❑ responsiveness of an instrument to changes over time

Cont'd

Table 8.3 Cont'd   Checklist for designing or reviewing a methodology study

---

Methods—give details of the following:
- ❏ potential risks and benefits
- ❏ feasibility of methods
- ❏ development of questionnaires
- ❏ timetable for data collection
- ❏ pilot study and how the pilot study data will be used

Reducing bias—describe:
- ❏ the blinding procedures
- ❏ the randomisation method for ordering the tests
- ❏ standardisation of conditions
- ❏ appropriateness of time between measurements

Statistical methods—give details of:
- ❏ the statistical method used to test each aim or hypothesis
- ❏ how the results of each data analysis will be interpreted
- ❏ the use of measurements not related to aims or hypotheses

---

Clinical studies

Experimental clinical studies are conducted to establish the equivalence, efficacy or effectiveness of new treatments or other health care practices in subjects who have an established illness. Alternatively, non-experimental studies can be used to assess whether subjects with disease (cases) have been exposed to different environmental factors than subjects who do not have the disease (controls). Whatever the study design, only the studies that are conducted with a high degree of scientific merit can lead to improved health care. Clearly, to achieve this, the effects of treatments and of confounders and environmental factors must be measured with both accuracy and precision.

In clinical trials and case-control studies, the selection of the subjects will have profound effects on the generalisability of the results. In both randomised and non-randomised clinical trials, it is vital that attention is given to improving subject compliance, to eliminating or reducing the effects of bias, and to minimising the effects of confounders. If data are being collected at more than one site, a management structure is needed to ensure quality control at all collection centres. A checklist for clinical studies that is supplemental to the core checklist (Table 8.2) is shown in Table 8.4.

Table 8.4   Checklist for designing or reviewing a clinical study

Study design—describe in detail:
- ❏ whether efficacy, equivalence or effectiveness is being measured
- ❏ the defining characteristics of the subjects
- ❏ any matching strategies that will be used

Treatment or intervention—give details of:
- ❏ the placebo or control group treatment
- ❏ methods to assess short-term and long-term effects
- ❏ methods for measuring compliance
- ❏ the evaluation of potential risks

Methods—describe:
- ❏ the sampling methods
- ❏ ability to recruit the required number of subjects
- ❏ feasibility of data collection methods
- ❏ how the response rate will be maximised
- ❏ the questionnaires to be used
- ❏ the subjective, objective and surrogate outcome variables
- ❏ the methods to measure outcomes, such as quality of life, that are important to the patient
- ❏ the pilot study and how pilot data will be used
- ❏ a time-line to completion of the study
- ❏ feedback to subjects

Validity of measurements—give information of:
- ❏ repeatability of outcome and exposure measurements
- ❏ responsiveness of outcome measurements to change
- ❏ criterion or construct validity of measurements
- ❏ applicability of measurements to the aims of this study

Reducing bias and confounding—say how you will manage:
- ❏ selection bias
- ❏ observer bias and any blinding procedures
- ❏ follow-up procedures
- ❏ balancing confounders and prognostic factors
- ❏ randomisation of subjects to groups and allocation concealment

Statistical methods—give details of:
- ❏ the inclusion criteria for each analysis (intention to treat, selection, etc.)
- ❏ the statistical method used to test each hypothesis
- ❏ how any stratified analyses will be conducted
- ❏ how the results of each data analysis will be interpreted
- ❏ whether the sample size will allow a clinically important difference between study groups to be statistically significant
- ❏ how data not related to study aims will be used
- ❏ how threshold or dose–response effects will be assessed

Epidemiological studies

Epidemiological studies can be used for many purposes, including the measurement of estimates of incidence and prevalence, the quantification of risk factors, and the effects of environmental interventions. In such studies, the measurements of disease and exposure must be as precise as possible, and the sampling strategies must be designed to minimise bias and to maximise generalisability. In addition, sample size is a fundamental issue because many epidemiological studies are designed to make comparisons between populations or over time or between subgroups of the population, for which a large sample size is usually required. The way in which the study is designed will inevitably influence the extent to which populations or subgroups can be reliably compared, and the extent to which causation can be inferred from the identification of apparent risk factors.

The many issues that influence the generalisability and the precision of the results obtained from conducting a study of a population sample of subjects are shown in Table 8.5. This checklist is supplemental to the core checklist shown in Table 8.2.

Table 8.5 Checklist for designing or reviewing an epidemiological study

Study design—describe whether this study is:
- ❑ an ecological study
- ❑ a cross-sectional study (to measure prevalence, incidence, risk factors)
- ❑ a case-control or cohort study (to measure risk factors, prognosis)
- ❑ a population intervention (to measure effectiveness)

Subjects—give details of:
- ❑ how the subjects will be recruited
- ❑ whether a cohort is an inception or birth cohort
- ❑ whether only subjects with a disease of interest will be included
- ❑ the methods of random sampling

Methods—outline in detail:
- ❑ the feasibility of study
- ❑ the definitions used to identify the disease of interest
- ❑ measurement of confounders
- ❑ the pilot study and how the data will be used
- ❑ time-line for events
- ❑ feedback to subjects or community

Measurements—describe for the exposure and outcome measurements:
- ❑ repeatability
- ❑ criterion or construct validity
- ❑ applicability to this study

Cont'd

Table 8.5 Cont'd   Checklist for designing or reviewing an epidemiological
study

Reducing bias and confounding—describe how you will:
❑ maximise the response rate
❑ improve follow-up procedures
❑ assess non-responders to measure potential bias
❑ reduce observer bias
❑ measure and control for confounders
Statistical methods—give details of:
❑ the statistical method used to test each hypothesis
❑ how the results of each data analysis will be interpreted
❑ use of data not related to study aims
❑ methods to assess threshold or dose–response effects
❑ implications for causation

Section 2—Grantsmanship

The objectives of this section are to understand:
- how to prepare a competitive funding application;
- the importance of a team approach; and
- how to combine good science with excellent presentation.

Attracting research funding

Having a good idea for a study is an exhilarating moment in research, but obtaining funding to undertake the study is a daunting task. To attract funding, the study needs to be an innovative and achievable project that uses good science to produce clinically relevant information. For this, the study must be scientific, practical and likely to succeed, and the application must be beautifully thought out and superbly presented. The features that contribute to a successful application are shown in Table 8.6.

In contrast to the excitement of having a good idea for a study, developing the study design and completing the application forms is usually an endurance task that ensures that only the most dedicated will succeed. In addition to the knowledge needed to design a scientifically rigorous project, many other resources are required of which team support, time, peer review, patience and a competitive nature are essential. It is vital to be well organised because grant deadlines are not flexible. However, by planning a clear strategy, the chances of success can be maximised.[2]

Few researchers prepare a successful application all by themselves—a team approach is usually essential. Once a research idea has been translated into a testable hypothesis, the study design has been decided and the ideas are beginning to be documented, then it is time to consider a team approach to the paper work. It is enormously helpful if one person prepares the 'front-and-back' pages of a grant application—that is the budget, the principal investigators' bibliographies, the ethics applications, the signature

Table 8.6   Features of successful grant applications
Study design • based on novel ideas and good science • has clear relevance to evidence-based practice • designed to answer an important question • practical and likely to succeed • good value for money
Application • beautifully thought out • nicely presented • readable and visually attractive • well ordered

pages and so on. In this way, the principal investigators can focus on the science and the presentation with the confidence that someone else is taking responsibility for the clerical process.

To maximise the chances of being awarded a grant, you have to prepare one of the best applications in the granting round. This takes time—in fact, an amazing amount of time. Time is needed to work through and develop the study design, to get meaningful and ongoing peer review and feedback, and to take it on board and process it. It also takes a lot of time to edit and process many drafts. Only the allocation of sufficient resources will ensure that an application is both brilliantly thought out and perfectly presented.

It is prudent to remember that it is more ethical and more satisfying to design a study that uses the best science available, and that studies designed in this way also contribute to the research reputations of the investigators. Furthermore, this type of study is far more likely to attract funding. The benefit of all of this work is that striving for high marks will maximise the chances that the highest level of evidence will be collected in order to answer the study question. This is the only level of evidence that can contribute to the processes of evidence-based practice.

Peer review

The corner-stone of good science is peer review. When writing a funding application, it is important to elicit as much internal and external peer review as possible. This will ensure that the project becomes feasible and scientifically rigorous, uses the best study design to answer the research question, and has departmental support. Ideal people to ask are those who have been involved in research and have held a grant themselves, or have first-hand knowledge of the granting process. It is also essential to get feedback from 'outsiders'—for this, colleagues who work in a different research field and friends or family are ideal. If the application can be understood by people who are not research experts, then it stands a good chance of being easily understood by everyone involved in the peer review and granting processes.

It is a good idea to start as early as possible and to be realistic in allowing plenty of time for ideas to develop and for others to read the proposal, digest the concepts and give useful feedback. However, the very process of peer review can be both helpful and frustrating. Asking for advice from many quarters always elicits a wide diversity of opinions. When receiving peer review, the practical advice needs to be sifted out from the impractical advice, the scientific suggestions from the unscientific suggestions, and the personal agendas from your own agenda.

When receiving feedback, it can be dispiriting to have someone revise text that has taken many hours to compose, or suggest new ideas for a study that you have spent long hours designing. Nevertheless, for success, it is better to stand back and consider that if your peers have problems following your writing and understanding your rationale, then the granting committee will also have problems.

Presentation

Applications that are based on novel ideas, answer an important question, use good science and are value for money are prime candidates for funding. In addition, applications that are well thought out, readable and visually attractive are more likely to appeal to committee members who may not be content experts in your particular field.

Grantsmanship is a competitive process because only the applications with the highest marks are assured of success. Being competitive involves being prepared to edit many drafts in order to improve clarity and ensure a logical flow of ideas. It is a good idea to include diagrams, figures, tables and schematic time-lines to enable reviewers to grasp ideas at a glance. Paying attention to detail in the application signals to the committee that you are the type of person who will pay attention to detail when running the study.

For readability, be sure to use a topic sentence at the top of each paragraph. Also, delete the redundant phrases and sentences, use a large font and lots of white space, and avoid long words, abbreviations and adjectives. Be straightforward and substitute simple language such as 'is' instead of 'has been found to be', and direct terms such as 'will measure' instead of 'intends to detect' or 'aims to explore'. Remember that each of the reviewers and committee members have to process a large number of applications. It is inevitable that the applications that are a pleasure to read will be viewed more favourably.

Granting process

Essentially, only a handful of key readers will review an application in detail, that is the external reviewers who are content experts, and the granting committee, especially your spokesperson. These people, who have the responsibility of reading your protocol carefully, have a profound influence on whether your study is presented favourably to the rest of the committee. For this, the application needs to present good science packaged in such a way that it can be clearly and easily understood by the remainder of the committee who may not have had time to read it in depth. Remember that these people may not be experts in your research area.

Also, the committee members will be faced with a limited budget and a pile of applications—inevitably, their job is to avoid funding the majority of the applications before them. The committee will focus on any potential flaws in the logic and the study design, any problems that are likely to arise when conducting the study, and any better ways in which the research question could be answered. A good application addresses any limitations in the study design and gives clear reasons for the plan of action. The committee must also be convinced that the resources and expertise needed to bring the study to a successful conclusion will be available. Pilot data is very useful in this context. Conveying a sense of importance of the research topic and enthusiasm of the researchers will help too.

Justifying the budget

Finally, make sure that the budget is itemised in detail and is realistic. Unit costs and exact totals should be calculated. Budgets with everything rounded to the nearest $100 or $1000 not only suggest that they have been 'best guessed' but also suggest inattention to accuracy. Each item in the budget may need to be justified, especially if it is expensive and a cheaper alternative could be suggested. The cost benefits to the project of employing senior, and therefore more expensive, researchers rather than less experienced junior staff will also need to be made clear.

Research rewards

Most research requires a great deal of dedication to design the study, obtain the funding, recruit the subjects, collect and analyse the information, and report the data. However, there are some important events that make it all worthwhile, such as presenting an abstract at a scientific meeting, having an article published in a prestigious journal or having your results incorporated into current practice. One of the best rewards of all is obtaining a competitive funding grant. This always calls for celebration because it means that you have been awarded an opportunity to answer an important research question. This also means that the funding is deserved because a high quality application has been prepared for a study that plans to use the best science available to help improve health care.

Section 3—Research ethics

The objectives of this section are to understand:
- why ethical approval needs to be obtained;
- the issues that need to be considered in designing an ethical study; and
- research situations that may be unethical.

Ethics in human research

Ethical research always places the welfare and rights of the subject above the needs of the investigator. An important concept of research ethics is that a research study is only admissible when the information that will be collected cannot be obtained by any other means. Obviously, if it becomes clear during the course of a study that the treatment or intervention that is being investigated is harmful to some subjects, then the study must be stopped or modified. The ethical principles of research, which are widely published by governments and national funding bodies, are summarised in brief in Table 8.7.

Table 8.7   Ethical principles of research
• all research should be approved by an appropriate ethics committee
• the study findings will justify any risk or inconvenience to the subjects
• researchers should be fully informed of the purpose of the study and must have the qualifications, training and competence to conduct the study with a high degree of scientific integrity
• subjects must be free to withdraw consent at any time, and withdrawal must not influence their future treatment
• the rights and feelings of subjects must be respected at all times
• subjects must be provided with information on the purpose, requirements and demands of the protocol prior to their giving consent

Health science research

There are special ethical considerations when studying vulnerable people or populations.[3] There are also special considerations that relate to the study of children, the mentally ill, and unconscious or critically ill patients who are not empowered to give consent for study themselves. When conducting research in children, consent should be obtained from the parent or guardian in all but the most exceptional circumstances, and also from the child themselves when they reach sufficient maturity.[4]

The problems that arise from paying subjects to take part in research studies have been widely debated. In principle, subjects can be reimbursed for inconvenience and their time and travel costs but should not be induced to participate. Subjects should never be coerced into taking part in a research study and, for this reason, it is unethical to recruit subjects from groups such as friends, family or employees who do not feel that they have the freedom to refuse consent.

Ethics committees

Because almost all health care research is intrusive, it is essential that ethical approval is obtained from the appropriate local ethics committees. Members of ethics committees generally include a selection of people who provide a collective wide experience and expertise. Ethics committees often include laypersons, ministers of religion, lawyers, researchers and clinicians. The process of having the committee scrutinise each research study ensures that subjects are not placed under undue risk or undue stress. The process also ensures that the subjects will be fully informed of the purposes of the study and of what will be expected of them before they consent to take part. The responsibilities of ethics committees are shown in Table 8.8.

Table 8.8   Responsibilities of ethics committees

Ethics committees are convened to:
- protect the rights and welfare of research subjects
- determine whether the potential benefits to clinical practice in the long term warrant the risks to the subjects
- ensure that informed consent is obtained
- prevent unscientific or unethical research

It is widely accepted that clinical trials of new treatments or interventions are only ethical when the medical community is genuinely uncertain about which treatment is most effective. This is described as being in a situation of equipoise, that is uncertainty about which of the trial treatments would be most appropriate for the particular patient.[5] When patients are enrolled in clinical trials, there should always be concern about whether the trial is ethical because patients are often asked to sacrifice their own interests for the benefit of future patients. However, in practice, patients may participate in clinical trials out of self-interest and doctors may enter patients who have a personal preference for one of the treatments, which suggests that researchers and practitioners may have different attitudes to ethically acceptable practices.[6]

Unethical research situations

In research studies, situations that may be considered unethical sometimes occur. Because these situations usually occur inadvertently, it is always a good idea to consider the risks and benefits of a study from the subjects' perspectives and balance the need to answer a research question with the best interests of the study subjects. A list of some common potentially unethical situations is shown in Table 8.9.

Table 8.9   Research situations that may be unethical

Study design
- conducting research in children or disadvantaged groups if the question could be answered by adults
- using a placebo rather than standard treatment for the control group
- conducting a clinical study without an adequate control group
- any deviations from the study protocol
- beginning a new study without analysing data of the same topic from previous studies
- conducting studies of mechanisms that have no immediate impact on better health care

Research methods
- inclusion of questionnaires or measurements not specified in the ethics application
- enrolment of too few subjects to provide adequate statistical power
- stopping a study before the planned study sample has been recruited

Data analysis and reporting
- failure to analyse the data collected
- failure to report research results in a timely manner

Care of research subjects

In endeavouring to collect the 'best' available evidence about health care, it is important that the design of research studies is based on sound scientific principles to ensure that definitive conclusions will be obtained. It is also important that the selection of the subjects, the way in which consent is obtained, the manner in which trials are stopped, and the continuing care of the subjects are all considered.[7] In essence, all issues that relate to the care and respect of the subjects are a fundamental aspect of ethical research studies.

References

Introduction

1. Carpenter LM., Is the study worth doing? Lancet 1993; 342:221–223.

Chapter 1

1. Liddle J, Williamson M, Irwig L. Method for evaluating research and guideline evidence. NSW Department of Health. State Health Publication No 96-204 1996; pp 9–27.
2. Fowkes FGR, Fulton PM. Critical appraisal of published research: introductory guidelines. Br Med J 1991; 302:1136–1140.
3. Moyer VA. Confusing conclusions and the clinician: an approach to evaluating case-control studies. J Pediatrics 1994; 124:671–674.
4. Oxman AD, Sackett DL, Guyatt GH. Users' guide to the medical literature. I. How to get started. JAMA 1993; 270:2093–2095.
5. Guyatt GH, Sackett DL, Cook DJ. Users' guide to the medical literature. II. How to use an article about therapy or prevention. A. Are the results valid? JAMA 1993; 270:2598–2601.
6. Laupacis A, Wells G, Richardson S, Tugwell P. Users' guide to the medical literature. V. How to use an article about prognosis. JAMA 1994; 272:234–237.
7. Rosenberg W, Donald A. Evidence-based medicine: an approach to clinical problem-solving. Br Med J 1995; 310:1122–1126.
8. Haynes RB, Sackett DL, Muir Gray JA, Cook DL, Guyatt GH. Transferring evidence from research into practice: 2. Getting the evidence straight. Evidence-based medicine 1997; 2:4–6.
9. Sackett D. Is the evidence from this randomized trial valid? In Evidence-based medicine: how to practice and teach evidence-based medicine. New York: Churchill Livingstone, 1997; 92–99.
10. Mulrow CD. Rationale for systematic reviews. Br Med J 1994; 309: 597–599.
11. Solomon MJ, McLeod RS. Surgery and the randomised controlled trial: past, present and future. Med J Aust 1998; 169:380–383.
12. Egger M, Davey Smith G. Phillips AN. Meta-analysis. Principles and procedures. Br Med J 1997; 315:1533–1537.
13. Egger M, Davey Smith G. Meta-analysis. Potentials and promise. Br Med J 1997; 315:1371–1374.
14. Irwig L. Systematic reviews (meta-analyses). In: Kerr C, Taylor R,

Heard G, eds. Handbook of public health methods. Sydney: McGraw Hill, 1998; pp 443–448.
15. Editorial. Cochrane's legacy. Lancet 1992; 340:1131–1132.
16. Roland M, Torgerson D. What outcomes should be measured? Br Med J 1998; 317:1075.
17. Fullerton-Smith I. How members of the Cochrane Collaboration prepare and maintain systematic reviews of the effects of health care. Evidence-based medicine 1995; 2:7–8.
18. Chalmers I, Dickersin K, Chalmers TC. Getting to grips with Archie Cochrane's agenda. Br Med J 1992; 305:786–787.
19. Sackett DL, Rosenberg WMC, Gray JAM, Haynes RB, Richardson WS. Evidence-based medicine: what it is and what it isn't. Br Med J 1996; 312:71–72.
20. Gilbert R, Logan S. Future prospects for evidence-based child health. Arch Dis Child 1996; 75:465–473.
21. Rosenberg W, Donald A. Evidence-based medicine: an approach to clinical problem-solving. Br Med J 1995; 310:1122–1126.
22. Sackett DL, Haynes RB. On the need for evidence-based medicine. Evidence-based medicine 1995; 1:5–6.
23. Haynes RB, Sackett DL, Gray JAM, Cook DJ, Guyatt GH. Transferring evidence from research into practice: I. The role of clinical care research evidence in clinical decisions. Evidence-based medicine 1996; 1:196–197.
24. Maynard A. Evidence-based medicine: an incomplete method for informing treatment choices. Lancet 1997; 349:126–128.
25. Gilbert R, Logan S. Future prospects for evidence-based child health. Arch Dis Child 1996; 75:465–473.
26. Kerridge I, Lowe M, Henry D. Ethics and evidence-based medicine. Br Med J 1998; 316:1151–1153.

Chapter 2

1. DerSimonian R, Levine RJ. Resolving discrepancies between a meta-analysis and a subsequent large controlled trial. JAMA 1999; 282:664–670.
2. Haynes B., Can it work? Does it work? Is it worth it? Br Med J 1999; 319:652–653.
3. ibid.
4. Roland M, Torgerson DJ. Understanding controlled trials. What are pragmatic trials? Br Med J 1998; 316:285.
5. Ebbutt AF, Frith L. Practical issues in equivalence trials. Stat Med 1998; 17:1691–1701.
6. Whitehead J. Sequential designs for equivalence studies. Stat Med 1996; 15:2703–2715.

7. Jones B, Jarvis P, Lewis JA, Ebbutt AF. Trials to assess equivalence: the importance of rigorous methods. Br Med J 1996; 313:36–39.
8. Lebel MH, Freij BJ, Syrogiannopoulos GA, et al. Dexamethasone therapy for bacterial meningitis. New Engl J Med 1988; 319:964–971.
9. Nishioka K, Yasueda H, Saito H. Preventive effect of bedding encasement with microfine fibers on mite sensitisation. J Allergy Clin Immunol 1998; 101:28–32.
10. Idris AH, McDermott MF, Raucci JC, Morrabel A, McGorray S, Hendeles L. Emergency department treatment of severe asthma. Metered-dose inhaler plus holding chamber is equivalent in effectiveness to nebulizer. Chest 1993; 103:665–672.
11. Black N. Why we need observational studies to evaluate the effectiveness of health care. Br Med J 1996; 312:1215–1218.
12. Altman DG, Dore CJ. Randomisation and baseline comparisons in clinical trials. Lancet 1990; 335:149–153.
13. Begg C, Cho M, Eastwood S, et al. Improving the quality of reporting of randomised controlled trials. The CONSORT statement. JAMA 1996; 276:637–639.
14. Altman DG. Better reporting of randomised controlled trials: the CONSORT statement. Br Med J 1996; 313:570–571.
15. Collier J. Confusion over use of placebos in clinical trials. Br Med J 1995; 311:821–822.
16. Aspinall RL, Goodman NW. Denial of effective treatment and poor quality of clinical information in placebo controlled trials of ondansetron for postoperative nausea and vomiting: a review of published studies. Br Med J 1995; 311:844–846.
17. Freedman B. Equipoise and the ethics of clinical research. New Engl J Med 1987; 317:141–145.
18. Rothman KJ. Placebo mania. Br Med J 1996; 313:3–4.
19. Edwards SJL, Lilford RJ, Hewison J. The ethics of randomised controlled trials from the perspectives of patients, the public, and healthcare professionals. Br Med J 1998; 317:1209–1212.
20. Collier J. Confusion over use of placebos in clinical trials. Br Med J 1995; 311:821–822.
21. Knorr B, Matz J, Bernstein JA, et al. for the Pediatric Montelukast Study Group. Montelukast for chronic asthma in 6- to 14-year-old children. JAMA 1998; 279:1181–1186.
22. Rothman KJ. Placebo mania. Br Med J 1996; 313:3–4.
23. ibid.
24. Tramer MR, Reynolds DJN, Moore RA, McQuay HJ. When placebo controlled trials are essential and equivalence trials are inadequate. Br Med J 1998; 317:875–880.
25. Britton J, Knox AJ. Duplicate publication, redundant publication, and disclosure of closely related articles. Thorax 1999; 54:378.

26. Laidlaw DAH, Harrad RA, Hopper CD, et al. Randomised trial of effectiveness of second eye cataract surgery. Lancet 1998; 352:925–929.
27. Sibbald B, Roberts C. Crossover trials. Br Med J 1998; 316:1719.
28. Senn SJ, Hilderbrand H. Crossover trials, degrees of freedom, the carryover problem and its dual. Stat Med 1991; 10:1361–1374.
29. Ellaway C, Williams K, Leonard H, Higgins G, Wilcken B, Christo-doulou J. Rett syndome: randomised controlled trial of L-carnitine. J Child Neurol 1999; 14:162–167.
30. Zelen M. Randomized consent designs for clinical trials: an update. Stat Med 1990; 9:645–656.
31. Torgenson DJ, Roland M. Understanding controlled trials. What is Zelen's design. Br Med J 1998; 316:606.
32. Gallo C, Perrone F, De Placido S, Giusti C. Informed versus randomised consent to clinical trials. Lancet 1995; 346:1060–1064.
33. Agertoft L, Pedersen S. Effects of long-term treatment with an inhaled corticosteroid on growth and pulmonary function in asthmatic children. Resp Med 1994; 88:373–381.
34. McKee M, Britton A, Black N, McPherson K, Sanderson C, Bain C. Interpreting the evidence: choosing between randomised and non-randomised studies. Br Med J 1999; 319:312–315.
35. ibid.
36. Torgerson DJ, Sibbald B. Understanding controlled trials. What is a patient preference trial? Br Med J 1998; 316:360.
37. Martinez FD, Wright AL, Taussig LM, Holberg CJ, Halonen M, Morgan WJ, The Group Health Associates. Asthma and wheezing in the first six years of life. New Engl J Med 1995; 332:133–138.
38. Lasky T, Stolley PD. Selection of cases and controls. Epidemiologic Reviews 1994; 16:6–17.
39. Wachholder S, Silverman DT, McLaughlin JK, Mandel JS. Selection of controls in case-control studies. II. Types of controls. Am J Epidemiol 1992; 135:1029–1041.
40. Golding J, Greenwood R, Birmingham K, Mott M. Childhood cancer, intramuscular vitamin K, and pethidine given during labour. Br Med J 1992; 305:341–346.
41. Ekelund H, Finnstrom O, Gunnarskog J, Kallen B, Larsson Y. Admin-istration of vitamin K to newborn infants and childhood cancer. Br Med J 1993; 307:89–91.
42. Badawi N, Kurinczuk JJ, Keogh JM, et al. Antepartum risk factors for newborn encephalopathy: the Western Australian case-control study. Br Med J 1998; 317:1549–1553.
43. Badawi N, Kurinczuk JJ, Keogh JM, et al. Intrapartum risk factors for newborn encephalopathy: the Western Australian case-control study. Br Med J 1998; 317:1554–1558.
44. Salonen JT, Tuomainen T-P, Nyyssonen K, Lakka H-M, Punnonen K.

Relation between iron stores and non-insulin dependent diabetes in men: case-control study. Br Med J 1998; 317:727.

45. Flanders WD, Austin H. Possibility of selection bias in matched case-control studies using friend controls. Am J Epidemiol 1986; 124: 150–153.

46. Wacholder S, Silverman DT, McLaughlin JK, Mandel JS. Selection of controls in case-control studies. III. Design options. Am J Epidemiol 1992; 135:1042–1050.

47. Grulich A. Analytic studies: cohort and case-control studies. In: Kerr C, Taylor R, Heard G, eds. Handbook of public health methods. Sydney: McGraw Hill, 1998: 107–116.

48. Halken S, Host A, Hansen LG, Osterballe O. Effect of an allergy prevention programme on incidence of atopic symptoms in infancy. A prospective study of 159 'high-risk' infants. Allergy 1992; 47: 545–553.

49. Evans SJW. Good surveys guide. Go for small random samples with high response rates. Br Med J 1991; 302:302–303.

50. Kaur B, Anderson HR, Austin J, et al. Prevalence of asthma symptoms, diagnosis, and treatment in 12–14 year old children across Great Britain (International Study of Asthma and Allergies in Childhood, ISAAC UK). Br Med J 1998; 316:118–124.

51. Ebrahim S, Davey Smith G. Ecological studies are a poor means of testing aetiological hypotheses. Br Med J 1998; 317:678.

52. Douglas AS, Helms PJ, Jolliffe IT. Seasonality of sudden infant death syndrome in mainland Britain and Ireland 1985–95. Arch Dis Child 1998; 79:269–270.

53. Butler CC, Pill R, Stott NCH. Qualitative study of patients' perceptions of doctors' advice to quit smoking: implications for opportunistic health promotion. Br Med J 1998; 316:1878–1881.

54. Schmerling A, Schattner P, Piterman L. Qualitative research in medical practice. Med J Aust 1993; 158:619–622.

55. Green J, Britten N. Qualitative research and evidence-based medicine. Br Med J 1998; 316:1230–1232.

56. Peat JK, Toelle BG, Nagy S. Qualitative research: a path to better health care. Med J Aust 1998; 169:1230–1232.

57. Grisso JA. Making comparisons. Lancet 1993; 342:157–158.

58. Ellaway C, Christodoulou J, Kamath R, Carpenter K, Wilcken B. The association of protein-losing enteropathy with cobolamin C defect. J Inher Metab Dis 1998; 21:17–22.

59. Mertens TE. Estimating the effects of misclassification. Lancet 1993; 342:418–420.

60. Barry D. Differential recall bias and spurious associations in case/control studies. Stat Med 1996; 15:2603–2616.

61. Fontham ET, Correa P, Reynolds P, et al. Environmental tobacco smoke

and lung cancer in nonsmoking women. A multicentre study. JAMA 1994; 271:1752–1759.

62. Barry D. Differential recall bias and spurious associations in case/control studies. Stat Med 1996; 15:2603–2616.

63. Evans SJW. Good surveys guide. Go for small random samples with high response rates. Br Med J 1991; 302:302–303.

64. Lavori PW, Louis TA, Bailar III JC, Polansky M. Designs for experiments—parallel comparisons of treatment. New Engl J Med 1983; 309:1291–1298.

65. Marcus SM. Assessing non-consent bias with parallel randomised and non-randomised clinical trials. J Clin Epidemiol 1997; 50:823–828.

66. Peat JK, Toelle BG, van den Berg R, Britton WJ, Woolcock AJ. Serum IgE levels, atopy, and asthma in young adults: results from a longitudinal cohort study. Allergy 1996; 51:804–810.

67. Bowler SD, Green A, Mitchell CA. Buteyko breathing techniques in asthma: a blinded randomised controlled study. Med J Aust 1998, 169: 575–578.

68. Hensley MJ, Gibson PG. Promoting evidence-based alternative medicine. Med J Aust 1998; 169:573–574.

69. Mertens TE. Estimating the effects of misclassification. Lancet 1993; 342:418–420.

70. Mayon-White RT. Assessing the effects of environmental pollution when people know that they have been exposed. Br Med J 1997; 314:343.

71. Chalmers TC, Celano P, Sacks HS, Smith H. Bias in treatment assignment in controlled clinical trials. New Engl J Med 1983; 309: 1358–1361.

72. Passaro KT, Noss J, Savitz DA, Little RE, The Alspac Study Team. Agreement between self and partner reports of paternal drinking and smoking. Int J Epidemiol 1997; 26:315–320.

73. Stern JM, Simes RJ. Publication bias: evidence of delayed publication in a cohort study of clinical research projects. Br Med J 1997; 315:640–645.

74. Tramer MR, Reynold DJM, Moore RA, McQuay HJ. Impact of covert duplicate publication on meta-analysis: a case study. Br Med J 1997; 315:635–640.

75. Egger M, Davey Smith G. Meta-analysis. Bias in location and selection of studies. Br Med J 1998; 316:61–66.

76. Egger M, Davey Smith G, Schneider M, Minder C. Bias in meta-analysis detected by a simple graphical test. Br Med J 1997; 315:629–634.

77. Choi PT, Yip G, Quinonez LG, Cook DJ. Crystalloids vs. colloids in fluid resuscitation: a systematic review. Crit Care Med 1999; 27: 200–210.

78. Marshall RJ. Assessment of exposure misclassification bias in case-control studies using validation data. J Clin Epidemiol 1997; 50:15–19.

79. Rowland ML, Forthofer RN. Adjusting for non-response bias in a health

examination survey. Public health reports 1993; 108:380–386.

80. Barry D. Differential recall bias and spurious associations in case/control studies. Stat Med 1996; 15:2603–2616.

81. Pocock SJ. Clinical trials. A practical approach. John Wiley and Sons Ltd, Somerset UK 1996; pp 90–99.

82. Schultz KF. Randomised trials, human nature, and reporting guidelines. Lancet 1996; 348:596–598.

83. Schultz KF. Subverting randomisation in controlled trials. JAMA 1995; 274:1456–1458.

84. Altman DG, Dore CJ. Randomisation and baseline comparisons in clinical trials. Lancet 1990; 335:149–153.

85. Sackett DL, Haynes RB, Guyatt GJ, Tugwell P. Clinical epidemiology. A basic science for clinical medicine. Little, Brown and Company, Boston 1991; pp 173–185.

Chapter 3

1. de Blic J, Thompson A. Short-term clinical measurements: acute severe episodes. Eur Respir J 1996; 9:4s–7s.

2. Hemmingway H, Stafford M, Stansfeld S, Shipley M, Marmot M. Is the SF-36 a valid measure of change in population health? Results from the Whitehall II study. Br Med J 1997; 315:1273–1279.

3. Wilson RW, Gieck JH, Gansneder BM, Perrin DH, Saliba EN, McCue FC. Reliability and responsiveness of disablement measures following acute ankle sprains among athletes. JOSPT 1998; 27: 348–355.

4. Guyatt G, Walter S, Norman G. Measuring change over time: assessing the usefulness of evaluative instruments. J Chron Dis 1987; 40:171–178.

5. Guyatt GH, Deyo RA, Charlson M, Levine MN, Mitchell A. Responsiveness and validity in health status measurement: a clarification. J Clin Epidemiol 1989; 42:403–408.

6. Guyatt GH, Juniper EF, Walter SD, Griffith LE, Goldstein RS. Interpreting treatment effects in randomised trials. Br Med J 1998; 316: 690–693.

7. Pocock SJ. Clinical trials with multiple outcomes: a statistical perspective on their design, analysis, and interpretation. Controlled Clin Trials 1997; 18:530–545.

8. Roland M, Torgerson D. What outcomes should be measured? Br Med J 1998; 317:1075.

9. Lebel MH, Freij BJ, Syrogiannopoulos GA, et al. Dexamethasone therapy for bacterial meningitis. New Engl J Med 1988; 319:964–971.

10. Littenberg B. Aminophylline treatment in severe, acute asthma. JAMA 1988; 259:1678–1684.

11. Wrenn K, Slovis CM, Murphy F, Greenberg RS. Aminophylline therapy

for acute bronchospastic disease in the emergency room. Ann Int Med 1991; 115:241–247.

12. Guyatt GH, Juniper EF, Walter SD, Griffith LE, Goldstein RS. Interpreting treatment effects in randomised trials. Br Med J 1998; 316: 690–693.

13. Bucher HC, Guyatt GH, Cook DJ, Holbrook A, McAlister FA, for the Evidence-Based Medicine Working Group. Users' guides to the medical literature. XIX Applying clinical trial results. A. How to use an article measuring the effect of an intervention on surrogate end points. JAMA 1999; 282:771–778.

14. Roland M, Torgerson D. What outcomes should be measured? Br Med J 1998; 317:1075.

15. Fleming RT, DeMets DL. Surrogate end points in clinical trials: are we being misled? Ann Intern Med 1996; 125:605–613.

16. Burke V, Gracey MP, Milligan RAK, Thompson C, Taggart AC, Beilin LJ. Parental smoking and risk factors for cardiovascular disease in 10–12 year old children. J Pediatr 1998; 133:206–213.

17. Datta M. You cannot exclude the explanation you have not considered. Lancet 1993; 342:345–347.

18. Leon DA. Failed or misleading adjustment for confounding. Lancet 1993; 342:479–481.

19. Willett WC, Green A, Stampfer MJ, et al. Relative and absolute excess risks of coronary heart disease among women who smoke cigarettes. N Engl J Med 1987; 317:1303–1309.

20. Simpson J, Berry G. Multiple linear regression. In: Kerr C, Taylor R, Heard G, eds. Handbook of public health methods. Sydney: McGraw Hill, 1998: 296–301.

21. Belousova EG, Haby MM, Xuan W, Peat JK. Factors that affect normal lung function in white Australian adults. Chest 1997; 112:1539–1546.

22. Goodwin LD. Changing concepts of measurement validity. J Nursing Education 1997; 36:102–107.

23. Reddell J, Ware S, Marks G, Salome C, Jenkins C, Woolcock A. Differences between asthma exacerbations and poor asthma control. Lancet 1999; 352:364–369.

24. Haftel AJ, Khan N, Lev R, Shonfeld N. Hanging leg weight—a rapid technique for estimating total body weight in pediatric resuscitation. Ann Emergency Med 1990; 19:63–66.

25. Lim LL, Dobbins T. Reproducibility of data collected by patient interview. Aust NZ J Public Health 1996; 20:517–520.

26. Kaur B, Anderson HR, Austin J, et al. Prevalence of asthma symptoms, diagnosis, and treatment in 12–14 year old children across Great Britain (International Study of Asthma and Allergies in Childhood, ISAAC UK). Br Med J 1998; 316:118–124.

27. de Marco R, Zanolin ME, Accordini S, et al., on behalf of the ECRHS.

A new questionnaire for the repeat of the first stage of the European Community Respiratory Health Survey: a pilot study. Eur Respir J 1999; 14:1044–1048.

28. Ellaway C, Williams K, Leonard H, Higgins G, Wilcken B, Christodoulou J. Rett syndome: randomised controlled trial of L-carnitine. J Child Neurol 1999; 14:162–167.

29. Salome CM, Xuan W, Gray EJ, Belousova E, Peat JK. Perception of airway narrowing in a general population sample. Eur Respir J 1997; 10: 1052–1058.

30. Stone DH. Design a questionnaire. Br Med J 1993; 307:1264–1266.

Chapter 4

1. Healy MJR. Distinguishing between 'no evidence of effect' and 'evidence of no effect' in randomised controlled trials and other comparisons. Arch Dis Child 1999; 80:210–213.

2. Campbell H, Surry SAM, Royle EM. A review of randomised controlled trials published in Archives of Disease in Childhood from 1982–1996. Arch Dis Child 1998; 79:192–197.

3. Halken S, Host A, Hansen LG, Osterballe O. Effect of an allergy prevention programme on incidence of atopic symptoms in infancy. A prospective study of 159 'high-risk' infants. Allergy 1992; 47:545–553.

4. Hanley JA, Lippman-Hand A. If nothing goes wrong, is everything all right? JAMA 1983; 249:1743–1745.

5. Bach LA, Sharpe K. Sample size for clinical and biological research. Aust NZ J Med 1989; 19:64–68.

6. Julious SA, Campbell MJ. Sample size calculations for paired or matched ordinal data. Stat Med 1998; 17:1635–1642.

7. Devine S, Smith JM. Estimating sample size for epidemiologic studies: the impact of ignoring exposure measurement uncertainty. Stat Med 1998; 17:1375–1389.

8. Drescher K, Timm J. The design of case-control studies: the effect of confounding on sample size requirements. Stat Med 1990; 9:765–776.

9. Hanley J, McNeil BJ. The meaning and use of the area under a receiver operating characteristic (ROC) curve. Radiology 1982; 143:29–36.

10. Norman GR, Streiner DL., Biostatistics. The bare essentials. Missouri: Mosby Year Book Inc, 1994; p 168.

11. Day SJ, Graham DF. Sample size and power for comparing two or more treatment groups in clinical trials. Br Med J 1989; 299:663–665.

12. Norman GR, Streiner DL. Biostatistics. The bare essentials. Mosby Year Book Inc, Missouri 1994; pp 70–71.

13. Norman GR, Streiner DL., Biostatistics. The bare essentials. Missouri: Mosby Year Book Inc, 1994; p 168.

14. Stevens JP. Power of the multivariate analysis of variance tests. Pyschological Bulletin 1980; 88:728–737.
15. Norman GR, Streiner DL. Biostatistics. The bare essentials. Mosby Year Book Inc, Missouri 1994; pp 108–118.
16. Hsieh FY, Bloch DA, Larsen MD. A simple method of sample size calculation for linear and logistic regression. Stat Med 1998; 17: 1623–1634.
17. Norman GR, Streiner DL. Biostatistics. The bare essentials. Mosby Year Book Inc, Missouri 1994; pp 182–195.
18. McPherson K. Sequential stopping rules in clinical trials. Stat Med 1990; 9:595–600.
19. Abrams KR. Monitoring randomised controlled trials. Br Med J 1998; 316:1183–1184.
20. Geller NL, Pocock SJ. Interim analyses in randomised clinical trials: ramifications and guidelines for practitioners. Biometrics 1987; 43: 213–223.
21. Sandvik L, Erikssen J, Mowinckel P, Rodland EA. A method for determining the size of internal pilot studies. Stat Med 1996; 15: 1587–1590.
22. Birkett MA, Day SJ. Internal pilot studies for estimating sample size. Stat Med 1994; 13:2455–2463.
23. Geller NL, Pocock SJ. Interim analyses in randomised clinical trials: ramifications and guidelines for practitioners. Biometrics 1987; 43: 213–223.
24. Pocock SJ. When to stop a clinical trial. Br Med J 1992; 305:235–240.
25. Pocock S, White I. Trials stopped early: too good to be true? Lancet 1999; 353:943–944.
26. Abrams KR. Monitoring randomised controlled trials. Br Med J 1998; 316:1183–1184.
27. Pocock SJ. When to stop a clinical trial. Br Med J 1992; 305:235–240.
28. Pocock SJ, Hughes MD., Practical problems in interim analyses, with particular regard to estimation. Controlled Clin Trials 1989; 10:209s–221s.
29. Abrams KR. Monitoring randomised controlled trials. Br Med J 1998; 316:1183–1184.
30. Pocock SJ. When to stop a clinical trial. Br Med J 1992; 305:235–240.
31. ibid.
32. Pocock SJ. Current issues in the design and interpretation of clinical trials. Br Med J 1985; 290:39–42.

Chapter 5

1. Farrell B. Efficient management of randomised controlled trials: nature or nurture. Br Med J 1998; 317:1236–1239.

2. Knatterud GL, Rockhold FW, George SL, et al. Guidelines for quality assurance in multicenter trials: a position paper. Controlled Clin Trials 1998; 19:477–493.
3. Facey KM, Lewis JA. The management of interim analyses in drug development. Stat Med 1998; 17:1801–1809.
4. Farrell B. Efficient management of randomised controlled trials: nature or nurture. Br Med J 1998; 317:1236–1239.
5. Altman DG. Randomisation. Br Med J 1991; 302:1481–1482.
6. Quinlan KP, Hayani KC. Vitamin A and respiratory syncytial virus infection. Arch Pediatr Adolesc Med 1996; 150:25–30.
7. ibid.
8. Altman DG, Bland JM. Treatment allocation in controlled trials: why randomise? Br Med J 1999; 318:1209.
9. Laidlaw DAH, Harrad RA, Hopper CD, et al. Randomised trial of effectiveness of second eye cataract surgery. Lancet 1998; 352:925–929.
10. Abel U. Modified replacement randomization. Stat Med 1987; 6: 127–135.
11. Pocock SJ. Methods of randomisation. In Clinical trials. A practical approach. Somerset UK: John Wiley & Sons Ltd, 1996; pp 66–89.
12. Treasure T, MacRae KD. Minimisation: the platinum standard for trials? Br Med J 1998; 317:362–363.
13. Pocock SJ. Methods of randomisation. In Clinical trials. A practical approach. Somerset UK: John Wiley & Sons Ltd, 1996; pp 66–89.
14. Signorini DF, Lueng O, Simes RJ, Beller E, Gebski VJ. Dynamic balanced randomisation for clinical trials. Stat Med 1993; 12: 2343–2350.
15. Pocock SJ. Clinical trials. A practical approach. Somerset UK: John Wiley & Sons Ltd, 1996; pp 87–89.
16. Chavasse DC, Shier RP, Murphy OA, Huttly SRA, Cousens SN, Akhtar T. Impact of fly control on childhood diarrhoea in Pakistan: community-randomised trial. Lancet 1999; 353:22–25.
17. Kerry SM, Bland JM. Trials which randomise practices I. How should they be analysed? Family Practice 1998; 15:80–83.

Chapter 6

1. Editorial. Subjectivity in data analysis. Lancet 1991; 337:401–402.
2. Rothman KJ. Modern epidemiology. Boston, Massachusetts: Little, Brown and Company, 1986; pp 147–150.
3. Michels KB, Rosner BA. Data trawling: to fish or not to fish. Lancet 1996; 348:1152–1153.
4. Savitz DA, Olshan AF. Multiple comparisons and related issues in the interpretation of epidemiologic data. Am J Epidemiol 1995; 142:904–908.
5. Altman DG, Bland JM. Detecting skewness from summary information. Br Med J 1996; 313:1200–1201.

6. Idris AH, McDermott MF, Raucci JC, Morrabel A, McGorray S, Hendeles L. Emergency department treatment of severe asthma. Metered-dose inhaler plus holding chamber is equivalent in effectiveness to nebulizer. Chest 1993; 103:665–672.
7. Gardner MJ, Gardner SB, Winter PD. Confidence interval analysis (CIA). BMJ Publishing Group, 1992.
8. Altman DG, Dore CJ. Randomisation and baseline comparisons in clinical trials. Lancet 1990; 335:149–153.
9. ibid.
10. Lebel MH, Freij BJ, Syrogiannopoulos GA, et al. Dexamethasone therapy for bacterial meningitis. New Engl J Med 1988; 319:964–971.
11. ibid.
12. Jolley D. The glitter of the t-table. Lancet 1993; 342:27–28.
13. Hollis S, Campbell F. What is meant by intention to treat analyses? Survey of published randomised controlled trials. Br Med J 1999; 319: 670–674.
14. Newell DJ. Intention-to-treat analysis: implications for quantitative and qualitative research. Int J Epidemiol 1992; 21:837–841.
15. ibid.
16. Pocock SJ, Abdalla M. The hopes and hazards of using compliance data in randomized controlled trials. Stat Med 1998; 17:303–317.
17. Rosman NP, Colton T, Labazzo J, et al. A controlled trial of diazepam administered during febrile illnesses to prevent recurrence of febrile seizures. N Engl J Med 1993; 329:79–84.

Chapter 7

1. Childs C, Goldring S, Tann W, Hiller VF. Suprasternal doppler ultrasound for assessment of stroke distance. Arch Dis Child 1998; 79: 251–255.
2. Bland JM, Altman DG. Statistical methods for assessing agreement between two methods of clinical measurement. Lancet 1986; 1: 307–310.
3. Bland JM, Altman DG. Measurement error and correlation coefficients. Br Med J 1996; 313:41–42.
4. Chinn S. Repeatability and method comparison. Thorax 1991; 46: 454–456.
5. Bland JM, Altman DG. Statistical methods for assessing agreement between two methods of clinical measurement. Lancet 1986; 1: 307–310.
6. Muller R, Buttner P. A critical discussion of intraclass correlation coefficients. Stat Med 1994; 13:2465–2476.
7. Altman DG, Bland JM. Comparing several groups using analysis of variance. Br Med J 1996; 312:1472–1473.

8. Armitage P, Berry G. Statistical methods in medical research. Blackwell Science, 1997; pp 273–276.
9. Shrout PE, Fleiss JL. Intraclass correlations: uses in assessing rater reliability. Psychol Bull 1979; 86:420–428.
10. Morton AP, Dobson AJ. Assessing agreement. Med J Aust 1989; 150: 384–387.
11. Chinn S, Burney PGJ. On measuring repeatability of data from self-administered questionnaires. Int J Epidemiol 1987; 16:121–127.
12. Bland JM, Altman DG. Statistical methods for assessing agreement between two methods of clinical measurement. Lancet 1986; 1: 307–310.
13. ibid.
14. Bland JM, Altman DG. Comparing methods of measurement: why plotting difference against standard method is misleading. Lancet 1995; 346:1085–1087.
15. Tanner M, Nagy S, Peat J. Detection of infants' heartbeat or pulse by parents: a comparison of four methods. J Paediatrics 2000; 137:429–430.
16. ibid.
17. Bland JM, Altman DG. Statistical methods for assessing agreement between two methods of clinical measurement. Lancet 1986; 1: 307–310.
18. Bland JM, Altman DG. Measurement error and correlation coefficients. Br Med J 1996; 313:41–42.
19. Bland JM, Altman DG. Measurement error. Br Med J 1996; 313:744.
20. Haftel AJ, Khan N, Lev R, Shonfeld N. Hanging leg weight—a rapid technique for estimating total body weight in pediatric resuscitation. Ann Emergency Med 1990; 19:63–66.
21. Bhutani VK, Johnson L, Sivieri EM. Predictive ability of a predischarge hour-specific serum bilirubin for subsequent significant hyperbilirubinemia in healthy term and near-term newborns. Pediatrics 1999; 103:6–14.
22. ibid.
23. Altman DG, Bland JM. Diagnostic tests 2: predictive values. Br Med J 1994; 309:102.
24. ibid.
25. ibid.
26. ibid.
27. Sackett DL, Straus S. On some clinically useful measures of the accuracy of diagnostic tests. Evidence-based medicine 1998; 3:68–70.
28. Gardner MJ, Gardner SB, Winter PD. Confidence interval analysis (CIA). BMJ Publishing Group 1992.
29. Altman DG, Bland JM. Diagnostic tests 3: receiver operating characteristics plots. Br Med J 1994; 309:188.
30. Bhutani VK, Johnson L, Sivieri EM. Predictive ability of a predischarge

hour-specific serum bilirubin for subsequent significant hyperbilirubinemia in healthy term and near-term newborns. Pediatrics 1999; 103:6–14.

31. Altman DG, Bland JM. Diagnostic tests 2: predictive values. Br Med J 1994; 309:102.
32. Hanley J, McNeil BJ. The meaning and use of the area under a receiver operating characteristic (ROC) curve. Radiology 1982; 143:29–36.
33. Zweig MH, Campbell G. Receiver-operating characteristic (ROC) plots: a fundamental tool in clinical medicine. Clin Chem 1993; 39: 561–577.
34. Li J, Peat JK, Xuan W, Berry G. Meta-analysis on the association between environmental tobacco smoke (ETS) exposure and the prevalence of lower respiratory tract infection in early childhood. Pediatric Pulmonology 1999; 27:5–13.
35. Deeks J. When can odds ratios mislead? Br Med J 1998; 317: 1155–1156.
36. Sackett D. Down with odds ratios! Evidence-Based Medicine 1996; 1: 164–166.
37. Zhang J, Yu KF. What's the relative risk? A method of correcting the odds ratio in cohort studies of common outcomes. JAMA 1998; 280: 1690–1691.
38. Sackett DL. On some clinically useful measures of the effects of treatment. Evidence-Based Medicine 1996; 1:37–38.
39. Altman DG. Confidence intervals for number needed to treat. Br Med J 1998; 317:1309–1312.
40. Guyatt GH. Users' guide to the medical literature. II. How to use an article about therapy or prevention. B. What were the results and will they help me in caring for my patients? JAMA 1994; 271: 59–63.
41. Cook RJ, Sackett DL. The number needed to treat: a clinically useful measure of treatment effect. Br Med J 1995; 310:452–454.
42. Gardner MJ, Gardner SB, Winter PD. Confidence interval analysis (CIA). BMJ Publishing Group 1992.
43. Cook RJ, Sackett DL. The number needed to treat: a clinically useful measure of treatment effect. Br Med J 1995; 310:452–454.
44. Altman DG. Confidence intervals for number needed to treat. Br Med J 1998; 317:1309–1312.
45. ibid.
46. Davidson RA. Does it work or not? Clinical vs statistical significance. Chest 1994; 106:932–934.
47. Hall SM, Glickman M. The British Paediatric Surveillance Unit. Arch Dis Child 1988; 63:344–346.
48. Elliott EJ, Chant KG. Rare disease surveillance. J Paediatr Child Health 1994; 30:463–465.

49. Simon R. A decade of progress in statistical methodology in clinical trials. Stat Med 1991; 10:1789–1817.
50. Royle JA, Williams K, Elliott E, et al. Kawasaki disease in Australia, 1993–95. Arch Dis Child 1998; 78: 33–39.
51. Australian Bureau of Statistics. Risk factors. National Health Survey. ABS Catalogue No. 4360.0 1995; pp 8–11.
52. ibid.
53. Royle JA, Williams K, Elliott E, et al. Kawasaki disease in Australia, 1993–95. Arch Dis Child 1998; 78: 33–39.

Chapter 8

1. Sitthi-amorn C, Poshyachinda V. Bias. Lancet 1993; 342:286–288.
2. Goldblatt D. How to get a grant funded. Br Med J 1998; 317:1647–1648.
3. Gostin L. Macro-ethical principles for the conduct of research on human subjects: population-based research and ethics. In: Bankowski Z, Bryant JH, Last JM, eds. Ethics and epidemiology: international guidelines. Council for International Organizations of Medical Sciences (CIOMS), 1993; pp 29–46.
4. Report on the ethics of research in children. Aust Paediatr J 1981; 17: 162.
5. Peto R, Baigent C. Trials: the next 50 years. Br Med J 1998; 317: 1170–1171.
6. Edwards SJL, Lilford RJ, Hewison J. The ethics of randomised controlled trials from the perspectives of patients, the public, and healthcare professionals. Br Med J 1998; 317:1209–1212.
7. Kerridge I, Lowe M, Henry D. Ethics and evidence-based medicine. Br Med J 1998; 316:1151–1153.

Index

*Pages followed by 'e' indicate examples; pages followed by 'f' indicate figures; pages followed by 't' indicate tables; glossary terms are in **bold**.*